D1558838

WITHDRAWN

Self-Assessment Color Review of
Avian Medicine

Robert B. Altman
DVM
Avian, Exotic and Surgical Consultants Inc.
Boca Raton, Florida, USA

Neil A. Forbes
BVetMed, CBiol, MIBiol, Dip ECAMS, FRCVS
RCVS & European Specialist in Avian Medicine and Surgery
Clock House Veterinary Hospital
Stroud, Gloucestershire, UK

Iowa State University Press/Ames

Acknowledgements

We wish to thank Manson Publishing for acting as the catalyst for this book. We thank our respective wives for their patience and support during the preparation of this book. Above all we thank the contributors for their time, experience, and for sharing their expertise.

Dedications

R.B.A.
To Etta, who's indomitable spirit has been an inspiration, and to my grandchildren Jessica, Joey, Jessica, Joshua, Jesse, Logan and Ethan.

N.F.
To Claire for her understanding during the preparation of this book and to my daughters Katy and Sarah-Jane.

R.B.A. and N.F.
To students of avian medicine and surgery, 'new, young and old' together with their long-suffering families and colleagues.

First published in the United States of America in 1998 by
Iowa State University Press, 2121 South State Avenue, Ames, Iowa 50014-8300.
ISBN 0–8138–2339–0
Library of Congress Cataloging-in-Publication Data applied for.

Editing: Peter H. Beynon
Typesetting, design and layout: Paul Bennett
Cover design: Patrick Daly
Color reproduction: Reed Digital, Ipswich, UK
Printed by: Grafos SA, Barcelona, Spain

Preface

As the result of the explosion of information disseminated over the past few years, avian patients are rapidly becoming a routine part of the case load seen by many clinicians. The level of expertise of those specializing in avian medicine has elevated along with the interest of veterinary clinicians and aviculturists, resulting in a demand for the practise of high-quality medicine.

There are many quality reference texts on avian medicine and surgery which offer detailed in-depth information; however, accessing this information can be laborious and time consuming. This book along with others in the series is designed to assess one's level of knowledge and offers comprehensive, clinically-oriented information that can be quickly accessed, easily understood and applied

The book covers a wide range of disciplines, organ systems and species but is not as all inclusive as a text would be. The questions are presented in the same way clinical cases would be presented on a daily basis, challenging the reader to real clinical situations and in most cases offering a comprehensive solution to the question.

The book is designed to be fun to read while at the same time being instructive. This type of learning has proven to be the most effective for neophyte avian practitioners as well as experienced clinicians by guiding the reader through the main decision-making processes.

In compiling this book we have enlisted contributions from leading international authorities with diverse fields of expertise. We are sure that there will be varying opinions on some of the material presented and that products discussed will not be available in all countries. To allow the inclusion of additional questions, referencing of the material presented was omitted because of space and cost constraints.

We hope that the reader will find this book a useful learning tool and at the same time enjoy the learning process.

Robert B. Altman
Neil A. Forbes
1998

Contributors

Robert B. Altman, DVM (Avian)
Exotic and Surgical Consultants Inc.,
Boca Raton, Florida, USA

John R. Baker, BVSc, PhD, FSA Scot,
    MIBiol, CBiol, MRCVS
Rhosesmor, Mold, Flintshire, UK

R. Avery Bennett, DVM, MS, Dip ACVS
Univerity of Florida, Gainesville, Florida,
USA

Terry W. Campbell, DVM, MS, PhD
Colorado State University, Fort Collins,
Colorado, USA

Susan L. Clubb, DVM, Dip ABVP (Avian)
Parrot Jungle and Gardens, Miami,
Florida, USA

Michelle Curtis Velasco, DVM, Dip AVBP
    (Avian)
Fleming Island Pet and Bird Clinic, Orange
Park, Florida, USA

Michael Doolen, DVM
Avian and Exotic Animal Hospital of
Oakhurst, Oakhurst, New Jersey, USA

Gerry M. Dorrestein, DipVetPath,
    Dip LabAnimPath
University of Utrecht, Utrecht,
The Netherlands

Neil A. Forbes, BVetMed, CBiol, MIBiol,
    Dip ECAMS, FRCVS
Clock House Veterinary Hospital, Stroud,
Gloucestershire, UK

Alan M. Fudge, DVM, Dip ABVP (Avian)
California Avian Laboratory/Avian
Medical Center of Sacramento, Citrus
Heights, California, USA

Nigel H. Harcourt-Brown, BVSc, FRCVS
Harrogate, North Yorkshire, UK

Manfred Hochleithner, DMV, Dip ECAMS
Tierklinik, Vienna, Austria

Jan Hooimeijer, DVM
Vogelkliniek Meppel, GM Meppel, The
Netherlands

Jeffrey R. Jenkins, DVM, Dip ABVP (Avian)
Avian and Exotic Animal Hospital,
San Diego, California, USA

Rüdiger Korbel, DVM, CertSAD,
    CertVOphthal, Dip ECAMS
University of Munich, Oberschleissheim,
Germany

Jerry LaBonde, DVM
Avian/Exotic Animal Hospital, Englewood,
Colorado, USA

Sjeng Lumeij, DVM, PhD, Dip ECAMS,
    Dip ABVP (Avian)
University of Utrecht, Utrecht,
The Netherlands

Glenn Olsen, DVM, MS, PhD
Patuxent Wildlife Research Center, Laurel,
Maryland, USA

Tomas W. Pennycott, BVMS, CertPMP
SAC Veterinary Services, Ayr, Ayrshire, UK

Tom Roudybush, BS, MS
Sacramento, California, USA

Jaime Samour, MVZ, PhD
National Avian Research Centre,
Abu Dhabi, UAE

Robert E. Schmidt, DVM, Dip ACVP
Zoo/Exotic Pathology Service,
West Sacramento, California, USA

Katja Trinkaus, DVM, DMV
Wartweg, Giessen, Germany

Thomas N. Tully, Jr., DVM, MS,
    Dip ABVP (Avian)
LSU School of Veeterinary Medicine,
Baton Rouge, Louisiana, USA

Margaret A. Wissman, DVM, Dip ABVP
    (Avian)
Icarus Mobile Veterinary Service, Wesley
Chapel, Florida, USA

Amy B. Worrell, BS Zoology, DVM,
    Dip ABVP (Avian)
All Pets Medical Center, West Hills,
California, USA

Classification of cases

Abbreviations

ACTH   adrenocorticotrophic hormone
ALAD   δ-aminolevulinic acid dehydrase
APA   air sac perfusion anaesthesia
AST   aspartate aminotransferase
b.i.d.   *bis in die* – twice a day
BMR   basal metabolic rate
BUN   blood urea nitrogen
CaEDTA   calcium disodium versonate
CBC   complete blood count
CITES   Convention on International Trade in Endangered Species (of Wild Fauna and Flora)
CK   creatine kinase
CNS   central nervous system
CPK   creatine phosphokinase
D   dioptre (unit of refracting power of lenses)
DDT   dichlorodiphenyltrichloroethane
DMSA   meso-2,3-dimercaptosuccinic acid
DNA   deoxyribonucleic acid
DVE   duck viral enteritis
DVH   duck viral hepatitis
ECG   electrocardiogram
EDTA   ethylenediaminetetraacetic acid
ELISA   enzyme-linked immunosorbent assay
FFA(s)   free fatty acid(s)
GI   gastrointestinal(ly)
Hb   haemoglobin
HCG   human chorionic gonadotropin
HCl   hydrochloric [acid/fumes]
HIV   human immunodeficiency virus
HLA   human lymphocyte antigens
IBH   inclusion body hepatitis
IFA   immunoflourescent antibodies
i.m.   intramuscular(ly)

IU   international unit
i.v.   intravenous(ly)
LDE   long digital extensor
LDH   lactate dehydrogenase
LRS   lactated Ringer's solution
MCHC   mean corpuscular haemoglobin concentration
MHz   megahertz
MIC   minimum inhibitory concentration
mV   millivolt
(P)BFD   (psittacine) beak and feather disease
PCR   polymerase chain reaction
PCV   packed cell volume
PEG   polyethylene glycol
p.o.   *per os* – by mouth
PMV   paramyxovirus
ppm   parts per million
psi   pounds per square inch
pu/pd   polyuria/polydipsia
RBC(s)   red blood cell(s)
s.c.   subcutaneous(ly)
SGOT   serum glutamic–oxaloacetic transaminase
s.i.d.   once a day
TIBC   total [serum] iron binding capacity
t.i.d.   *ter in die* – three times a day
TP   total protein
TPA   tissue plasminogen activator
UA   uric acid
UV   ultraviolet
UIBC   unsaturated iron binding capacity
WBC   white blood cell

1 Feathers are the most distinctive feature of avian anatomy (**1**).
i. What are the three main functions of feathers?
ii. Give a description of the function of the following feathers: flight feathers, down feathers, semiplumes, filoplumes and bristles.

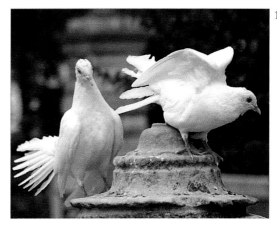

2 i. This endoscopic photograph (**2**) shows a large number of roundworms. Can you identify the anatomical site and the parasite in question? Is it:

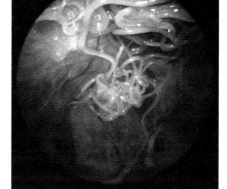

- *Syngamus trachea* in the crop of a bird?
- *Capillaria contorta* in the oesophagus of a bird?
- *Serratospiculum* sp. in the air sac of a bird?

ii. What percentage of wild saker (*Falco cherrug*), in their natural range countries, carry a burden of this parasite?
iii. Should such infections be treated and, if so, how?
iv. How are birds infected with this parasite?
v. How could a collection of birds be managed to prevent clinical disease caused by this parasite?

3 A ten-week-old cockatiel (post purchase from a pet shop) was examined. The veterinarian collected and submitted a screening blood panel. In addition to a monocytosis, salient clinical findings include the following details: AST (SGOT) 1450 IU/l (normal range 130–390 IU/l).
i. What organ is likely to be affected?
ii. How would you further characterize this insult?

1–3: Answers

1 i. Feathers are unique structures of the skin that provide insulation for controlling body temperature, aerodynamic power for flight and colours for communication and camouflage. Feathers also perform secondary roles. Modified feathers are important in swimming, sound production, hearing, protection, cleanliness, water repelling, water transport and tactile sensation.

ii. The flight feathers of the tail attach to the pygostyle and function primarily in steering and braking during flight.

Down feathers have loosely entangled barbules that trap air in a layer close to the skin, providing an excellent natural, lightweight thermal insulation. Powderdowns assist in cleaning the plumage.

Semiplumes enhance thermal insulation, fill out the aerodynamic contours of body plumage and serve as courtship ornaments.

Filoplumes are hairlike feathers that monitor the movement and position of adjacent veined feathers aiding aerodynamic adjustments.

Bristles are specialized feathers with both sensory and protective functions, e.g. eyelashes of ostriches or facial feathers of raptors.

2 i. *Serratospiculum* sp. is a large filarial worm found within the air sac walls, visceral membranous serosa and the connective tissue of the coeliomic cavity of raptors. **2** is from the air sac of a Gyr falcon (*Falco rusticolus*), which displayed laborious breathing and poor flight performance.

ii. Studies in central Asia suggest that up to 10–15% of the wild saker population are infected with *Serratospiculum* sp. Wild prairie falcons (*Falco mexicanus*) are also commonly affected in the USA.

iii. Current treatment for *Serratospiculum* sp. infections include ivermectin i.m. 0.2 mg kg^{-1} every week for 3 weeks or mebendazole p.o. 25 mg kg^{-1} daily for 2 weeks. Many clinicians believe that dead worms should be removed from the coeliomic cavity, using endoscopy following treatment, in heavily infected birds.

iv. The life cycle of *Serratospiculum* sp. is currently unknown. *S. tendo* is probably transmitted by the ingestion of *Locusta migratoria* containing infected larvae. Other species are probably transmitted by blood-sucking arthropods.

v. Although very little is known about the life cycle, it is highly recommended to control all ectoparasites on the birds and in their environment. Quarantine of newly imported birds, and isolation and treatment of infected birds, coupled with ectoparasite treatment, is recommended.

3 i. Similar to mammals, elevations in AST (SGOT) are non-specific. It is impossible to differentiate this elevation between hepatocellular leakage and damage from similar insults to cardiac, skeletal or smooth muscle. In this case, no venipuncture was performed, instead the sample had been collected from a nail clip.

ii. The enzyme CPK is of assistance in differentiating elevations. A patient presenting with an elevation of this enzyme – as well as AST (SGOT) – is less likely to be affected by hepatocellular damage or leakage.

4 Which of the following is correct? These oral lesions (4) in a juvenile cockatiel are most likely associated with:

- trichomoniasis;
- candidiasis;
- poxvirus infection;
- an accumulation of hand-rearing food.

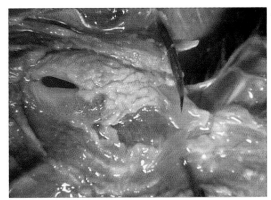

5 A six-year-old, yellow-naped Amazon parrot (5) is presented with blood in the droppings. On physical examination, no significant abnormalities are found. While discussing options with the owner, the bird has a seizure.
i. What is the most probable cause of the bird's problem?
ii. What diagnostics would be most appropriate?
iii. What treatment would be indicated?

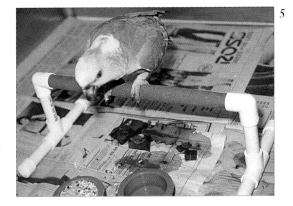

6 When a new toucan is purchased and in quarantine from the rest of the collection, prevention of transmittable diseases to the rest of the collection is of extreme importance.
i. What viral diseases should be considered?
ii. What bacterial diseases should be considered?
iii. What parasitic diseases should be considered?
iv. Are toucans susceptible to chlamydiosis?

4 These are lesions of oral candidiasis. It is a common problem in cockatiel chicks, both in the nest and chicks being handraised. It may also proliferate following antibiotic therapy.

5 i. Heavy metal poisoning, primarily lead. Clinical signs of lead toxicity are multi-systemic and involve depression, weakness, vomiting, pu/pd, seizures, haemoglobinuria and diarrhoea.
ii. Diagnostics would include a history of exposure to any sources of lead, radiographs, blood lead levels and haematology/blood chemistries. The absence of lead particles on radiographs does not rule out heavy metal toxicosis. Blood lead levels are acquired from whole blood in EDTA. Concentrations greater than 20 mg dl^{-1} (0.2 ppm) are suggestive, levels greater than 50 mg dl^{-1} (0.5 ppm) are diagnostic. ALAD and protoporphyrin concentrations may be used in confirming a diagnosis.
iii. Prior to running any diagnostics, the bird's seizures must be controlled, i.e. treat the patient not the toxin. If your suspicions are high for lead poisoning, chelation therapy may be commenced prior to laboratory confirmation. Therapy includes CaEDTA at 35 mg kg^{-1} i.m. b.i.d. until 48 hours after the cessation of clinical signs. Alternative oral chelation treatment for long-term therapy includes D-penicillamine – 55 mg kg^{-1} p.o. s.i.d. – or DMSA at 25–35 mg kg^{-1} daily for 5 days out of every 7 days for 3 weeks. Surgery to remove particulate lead is rarely indicated, however, if clinical signs reoccur or there are large pieces of lead present in the GI tract, then ventricular gavage under general anaesthetic will usually facilitate lead removal by a low-stress, non-invasive method.

6 i. To date, there are essentially no identified viral diseases that affect ramphastides. Thus, unlike psittacines, infectious and contagious viral diseases are not presently a concern in newly obtained toucans. Quarantine periods – extending a minimum of 6 weeks – are recommended for toucans, as for all avian species.
ii. Toucans are generally considered to be very hardy birds and do not contract many of the infectious diseases affecting other avian species. A small percentage of toucans develop upper respiratory infections that may be very difficult to completely clear. As with any type of animal with an upper respiratory infection, an affected toucan should be isolated from other birds. Quarantined toucans that develop such an infection should be treated accordingly. Toucans are reportedly considered to be highly susceptible to pseudotuberculosis, which is caused by the *Yersinia* sp. Thought to be transmitted by the ingestion of food contaminated by infected mice, this bacterial infection can be controlled by medication and management changes. Risk of bird-to-bird transmission is unlikely. Clinically affected toucans may die peracutely or demonstrate a chronic wasting.
iii. In the past – when importing toucans was common – a number of parasitic diseases were frequently diagnosed. These included coccidia, *Capillaria* sp., ascarids and *Giardia* sp. Any of these parasites could be potentially transmitted in a situation where access to another bird's droppings is possible.
iv. Ramphastides are potentially susceptible to infection with *Chlamydia psittaci* even though documented cases of ornithosis have not been identified in this type of bird.

7 The dark skin of this African grey parrot chick (7) is:
i. Normal pigmentation for this species.
ii. Indicates stunting and dehydration.
iii. Suggests that the chick is not actually an African grey parrot.
iv. Is only visible due to the lack of normal feathering.

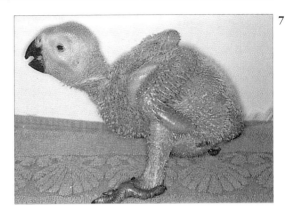

8 An African grey parrot is shown having a seizure, 'fitting', in 8.
i. List the main differential diagnoses and the causes of each one.
ii. Describe how you would reach your differential diagnoses.

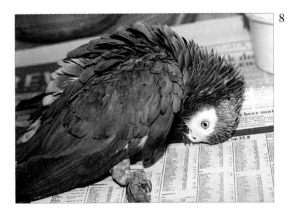

9 An eight-year-old red-breasted toucan (*Ramphastos tucanus*) (9) was presented for a post-mortem. The bird had been in the collection for 5 years; it was an aviary bird whose mate appeared healthy. The bird was clinically normal the previous day. On external examination, no abnormalities were noted and the body weight was considered good at 435 g.
i. What is the most likely diagnosis?
ii. What are the most likely gross post-mortem findings?

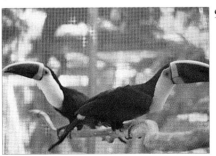

iii. What one specific tissue would be the most likely to demonstrate the cause of death?
iv. What other tissues might demonstrate characteristic changes in the bird?

7 The chick is normal.

8 i. The differential diagnoses are:

- Hypocalcaemia – this is particularly common in young (2–5-year-old) African grey parrots that have been fed on a poor, e.g. sunflower seed-based, diet These birds are deficient in Ca and vitamin D_3 or UV light. A viral condition affecting the parathyroid glands has also been implicated but to date has not been proven.
- Heavy metal poisoning – this is most commonly caused by lead or zinc and should be considered in any bird showing nervous signs. The signs demonstrated are dependent on the quantity of lead ingested and the chronicity of ingestion. Diagnosis comprises whole body radiography and blood lead analysis. Lack of radiographic evidence does not exclude lead poisoning. The diagnosis may be suspected if a dilated proventriculus and distal oesophagus is present. Non-enteric lead is generally considered to be non-pathogenic. Zinc poisoning most commonly occurs in new flights or aviaries, where galvanized wire, wire clips or other parts have been used. Poisoning is typically acute and metal particles are usually still evident on abdominal radiographs.
- Hypoglycaemia – this is caused by starvation, severely impaired liver function, infection or endocrine disorders.
- Hepatic encephalopathy – this is caused by any severe liver disease.
- Pesticide poisoning – this is caused by malicious or accidental poisoning through acetylcholinesterase inhibitors, e.g. carbamates, malathion, dichlorvos or organophosphates.
- Drug toxicities – e.g. dimetronidazole; levamisole.
- Meningitis – through bacterial, viral, parasitic or fungal infections.
- Idiopathic epilepsy.
- Trauma.

ii. Rapid diagnostic laboratory results are essential in cases involving fitting birds. A full haematology and biochemistry profile should be performed, as well as radiography and blood lead and zinc analysis. The most diagnostically important parameters are the haemogram (which may show evidence of infection), blood calcium and blood glucose levels.

9 i. The most likely diagnosis is iron storage disease (haemochromatosis). Cellular damage may or may not result from excessive iron deposition. Organ dysfunction and clinical illness or death may be the result. It is common to have a bird that appears clinically healthy prior to acute death.
ii. Hepatomegaly (often with a definite bronzed to bluish hue). Other organs are generally unremarkable.
iii. The liver is the predominant and frequently the only organ to be affected. Iron deposition can occasionally be noted in the spleen, kidney, lung, pancreas and intestine.
iv. Only rarely will iron pigment be identified in tissues other than the liver but these could include kidney, pancreas, intestine and lung, in that order of decreasing frequency of involvement.

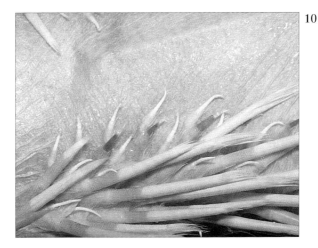

10

10 Gross appearance of feathers (**10**) from a young cockatoo that died following a short clinical illness.
i. What is the morphological diagnosis?
ii. What is the aetiological agent?
iii. What internal lesions would you expect?
iv. How can a definitive diagnosis be made?

11 'Pattern picking' – there are normal head feathers whilst only down feathers remain on the body (**11**). This is a clinically normal bird in all respects except for its plumage; all blood parameters are normal. Bacterial, fungal, parasitic, viral, chlamydial and metabolic aetiologies for feather plucking have been ruled out. The feathers on the head are totally normal. This bird was hand-reared and is now only 2 years old. The picking has been ongoing for 1 year. On occasion, during intimate 'cuddling sessions', the bird regurgitates on the owner. The bird only picks in the presence of the owner.
i. What is the likely cause of the picking?
ii. What are some of the treatment options?

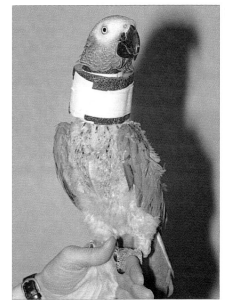

11

10 i. Multifocal follicular and feather pulp haemorrhage.

ii. These haemorrhages, which can vary in severity, are typical of polyomavirus infection in young psittacines.

iii. Depending on the species of psittacine, there is hepatic enlargement and variable necrosis, and splenomegaly. Generalized serosal haemorrhages may be present and, in a few cases, intestinal necrosis and haemorrhage are noted.

iv. Histologically, finding the characteristic lesions and inclusion bodies is diagnostic. Swabbing affected organs and submitting the swab for DNA probe testing is definitive, and, in cases with poorly developed lesions, may be the only way of making a positive diagnosis.

Cloacal swabs may be assessed by PCR for the presence of polyomavirus.

11 i. Reproductive hormonal pressure – sexual frustration – often begins to cause picking in young birds that are bonded to their owner even before reaching what is thought to be natural reproductive age. The hormonal drive provides a natural incentive for the young bird to try to achieve a status in the dominance hierarchy of the flock. This will lead to success in obtaining a mate, holding territory and having access to adequate food, so that it is able to reproduce. Captive birds often mature earlier than wild birds, especially when the owner is providing all the necessary advantages as well as stimulating it with a close bond. Consequently the bird reaches reproductive maturity but the 'mate' is not responding in the manner that will result in the production of offspring. This often leads to 'displacement behaviour' such as feather picking, screaming or aggression.

ii. Some success has been achieved with the administration of progesterones to decrease the hormonal pressure but some treated birds become obese, suffer from polyuria/polydipsia, diabetes mellitus or develop hepatic lipidosis. Recently, human chorionic gonadotrophin (HCG) (500–1000 IU kg^{-1} i.m.) has shown promise in providing effective, short-term resolution, especially in African grey parrots and cockatoo hens. There have been no reports of adverse reactions with this treatment but it is not always reliable. Tranquillizing agents – such as haloperidol – and psychotropic agents – such as clomipramine and Prozac – have shown some limited effectiveness in some individual cases. These medications can only provide a temporary solution and should be used in combination with behaviour modification techniques and changes in the bird's environment to provide a more reliable response. Petting on the bird's back and intimate cuddling should be reduced or eliminated.

For the owner to assert dominance the bird should be maintained below human chest height. The cage may be moved to a location away from the main traffic area to reduce the anxiety of seeing the owner without being cuddled. The length of the day may be shortened by covering the cage earlier in the evening and, in the case of females, surgical removal of the oviduct may provide the best long-term solution. In some cases, the picking becomes a habit, even though the original cause is resolved and long-term, anti-compulsive medication may be indicated.

12 This young, sulphur-crested cockatoo was recently purchased from a breeder with a PBFD-free, closed aviary and shipped by aeroplane to its new owner, who owns no other birds. The owner had saved up her money to purchase this one special bird as a pet. Being an informed and conscientious bird owner, she presents the bird to you for a complete health check, one week after its arrival at its new home. The bird looks perfectly normal on physical examination (**12**) and has completely normal feathers. Its weight is perfect for its size and it is bright, active and playful. The WBC count is, however, somewhat depressed (at 4.5×10^9 l^{-1}, 58% heterophils, 42% lymphocytes). You are surprised when the PBFD DNA PCR comes back positive (collected by a clean phlebotomy). What should you tell the owner?

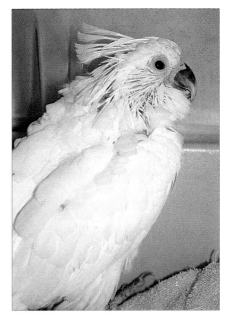

13 A male, four-year-old budgerigar, living in a flight cage with five other clinically normal birds, is presented with a powdery crust around the eyes, on the cere, in the intermandibular space, on the feet and around the vent (**13**). Skin scrapings confirm the presence of *Cnemidocoptes* sp. mites. In some cases the beak is rigid and overgrown. How should this case be managed?

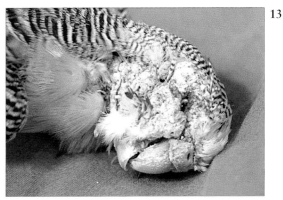

14 Which of the following is true? When treating the avian patient for hypovolaemia:

- Only crystalloid fluids – such as Ringer's solution or physiological saline – should be used.
- Only colloidal solutions – such as hetastarch or Dextran – should be used.
- Either crystalloid or colloidal solutions may be used; however, four times the volume of crystalloid solution is required to obtain the same effects.

12 A positive PBFD PCR in a young bird with no feather abnormalities suggests that the bird has recently been exposed to the virus and is currently viraemic or that it is latently infected. The best advice that can be given to the owner is not to panic as there is a good chance that the bird will be able to eliminate the virus on its own. If the bird was not shipped in a biosecure container, it may have been exposed to the virus en route in the cargo hold of the aircraft or at the airport, as circoviridae can generally remain viable in the environment for quite some time.

Blood for PBFD testing should be taken by clean venipuncture – and not a toe nail clip – as virus particles may otherwise contaminate the blood sample leading to a false positive.

Many young birds exposed to the virus will be transiently viraemic but will eliminate the virus. These birds will only develop disease if the immune system is unable to clear the infection. A PBFD-positive young bird with normal feathers should be kept isolated and retested in 90 days. If it is still positive it should be considered to be latently infected or that it is being continually exposed to the virus. A negative test after 90 days indicates that the bird has eliminated the infection. However, if a young bird is PBFD positive and has feather abnormalities, then the bird has active PBFD infection.

13 Treatment is simple and effective. Ivermectin – given orally at 0.2 mg kg^{-1} on two or three occasions at 2-week intervals – is effective. Infestation may be refractory in immunosuppressed birds.

The beak, if overgrown, may be shaped with a hand-held file or mechanical burr. If the germinal epithelial layer is damaged, the beak may continue to grow abnormally, even after the mites have been eradicated.

In affected adult birds immunosuppressive diseases must be considered, such as hepatic lipidosis, diabetes mellitus, or neoplasia. Since it is thought that there is some genetic disposition to this mite infestation, affected birds should not be used for breeding. All in-contact birds should also be treated in order to eradicate the parasite from the population as a whole.

14 The third choice is correct. Either crystalloid or colloidal fluids may be used to treat the hypovolaemic avian patient. Crystalloid fluids are highly effective at replacing fluids within the interstitial compartments, expanding circulating volume and enhancing diuresis; this facilitates the elimination of toxic by-products. These fluids rapidly leave the circulation and equilibrate in the interstitial fluid compartment. Only a quarter of isotonic fluids – such as LRS and 0.9% saline solution – remain in the vascular compartments of birds 30 minutes after administration. The infusion of large volumes of crystalloid fluids reduces colloid osmotic pressure and predisposes towards pulmonary and peripheral oedema, as well as predisposes to impaired peripheral tissue oxygen exchange. Synthetic colloids – hetastarch and dextrans – are polysaccharides of high molecular weight and particle size similar to albumen. The effect of their use is longer than crystalloids (24 hours in mammals). A dose of 10–20 ml kg^{-1} has been shown to be safe and efficacious in raptors and proven safe in clinical use.

15a

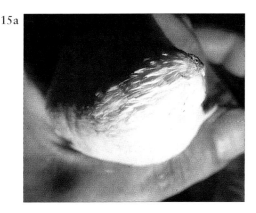

15b

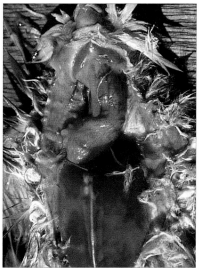

15c

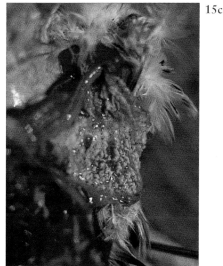

15 A budgerigar fancier says that some of his birds are vomiting; budgerigars flick their heads when vomiting with the result that some of the vomitus lands on the top of the head and causes matting of the feathers (15a). Some of the affected birds are dying. Post-mortem examination shows an enlarged and inflamed cranial oesophagus and proximal part of the crop (15b). On the crop mucosa there is an accumulation of yellow diphtheritic material (15c). What is the probable diagnosis? How might this diagnosis be confirmed?

16 i. Why are eggs stored before incubation?
ii. Under what conditions are eggs stored?
iii. What losses, if any, are expected?

17

15, 16: Answers

15 This will almost certainly be either trichomoniasis or candidiasis – both diseases produce the same symptoms and lesions. However, the former condition usually affects individual birds. Diagnosis depends on demonstrating the causal organism either in the lesions or in crop washes from live birds, although occasional false negatives are found with the latter method. As trichomonads die and disintegrate a few hours after the death of the bird, or after a crop wash is taken, only fresh samples are suitable for diagnosis of this disease. A wet film will show the highly motile trichomonads, and a Gram film or Diff Quik will show the yeast typical of *Candida* sp. The lesions of both diseases are heavily infiltrated with a mixed population of secondary bacteria.

In cases of trichomoniasis – because asymptomatic carriers will exist – all the birds on the premises should be treated. The usual treatment is dimetridazole in the drinking water. Care should be taken not to overdose as the margin of safety is not great. Signs of overdose are 'drunkenness' and incoordination followed by more severe signs of CNS disturbance, collapse and death. Other drugs that can be used for treatment are roni-dazole, carnidazole and metronidazole; it is not usually necessary to treat the secondary bacteria in cases of trichomoniasis. The treatment of individual birds with candida in-fections should include an antifungal agent, such as nystatin (300 000 IU kg^{-1} b.i.d. p.o. for 10 days).

16 i. In many species of birds the parents do not begin incubation until the entire clutch is laid. This helps to synchronize hatching. In captivity, it is often desirable, for manage-ment purposes, to synchronize the hatching of eggs, especially if nestlings are to be raised together and a larger, older nestling would pose a threat to smaller nestlings.
ii. The recommended conditions under which to store eggs are 12.8–18.3°C (55–65°F) though the low end of this range works best for most species. Relative humidity in the egg storage chamber should be 75%. Warming stored eggs once daily, to 27°C (80°F) for 5 minutes, helps to improve hatchability. Also, turning each egg 90° once daily, at the time of warming, improves embryo survival.
iii. Even under these optimal conditions, one can expect 2% per day loss of viable eggs – in 100 fertile eggs, two embryos will die off for each day of storage. Usually eggs are not stored for longer than 1 week as the loss of viable embryos may increase. Some non-domestic species, in particular passerine eggs, do not store well and this technique is not recommended. By contrast, waterfowl eggs generally do well when stored.

17 Radiograph (**17**) shows the ulna and radius of a Harris hawk, 3 weeks following repair of a compound fracture. The fracture is stable but the healing is not normal and the flight capability is impaired.

i. Describe the two pathological conditions shown in the illustration that might prevent a return to normal flight.

ii. Describe the advised treatment of each condition.

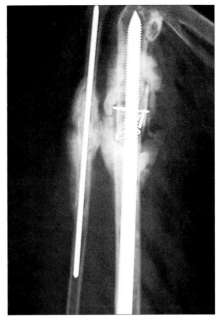

18 Three pheasants, aged eight weeks, were submitted alive with a flock history of loss of weight, diarrhoea and increased mortality. Following euthanasia, two of the birds were found to have frothy fluid-filled caecal contents and, in third bird (**18**), the caeca contained white casts. Wet preparations from all three birds demonstrated large numbers of motile protozoa measuring approx. 10 × 5 mm, each with a prominent undulating membrane.

i. What is the diagnosis?

ii. How is this condition treated and controlled?

iii. What other conditions can result in white caecal casts in pheasants?

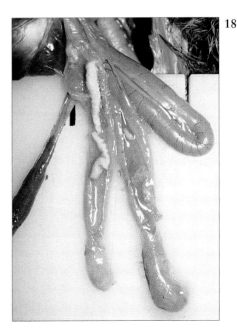

17, 18: Answers

17 i. The radiograph shows an active osteomyelitis with the presence of a bone sequestrum, as well as a synostosis between the radius and ulna.
ii. The bird should be anaesthetized, the pins and wire removed, and swabs taken for microbiology and sensitivity testing. The bird should receive systemic antibiotics; antibiotic-impregnated methylmethacrylate beads may be implanted at the site of the infection. These beads are effective in releasing antibiotic at the site of infection for a prolonged period of time. Once the infection is controlled, and the bone callous has fined down, a compressed air drill should be used to remove the synostosis that is currently fixing the ulna and radius in relation to each other. Such fixation of these bones prevents normal wing action. A fat pad should be placed between the radius and ulna at the site of the surgery in an attempt to prevent synostosis reformation. After one week's rest, to allow reduction of inflammation following surgery, the bird should be encouraged to keep the wing mobile.

18 i. The condition is trichomoniasis, caused by heavy burdens of *Trichomonas phasiani*. These motile protozoa are parasites of the caeca, causing problems in pheasants and partridges in rearing and release pens, and after release. Affected birds become lethargic with reduced appetite and weight loss, with arched backs and drooping wings. The caecal droppings of such birds are often yellow or orange and appear frothy. Many gamebirds are carriers, disease being precipitated by stress, over-crowding, poor hygiene, etc. Carcasses are dehydrated and thin, the caeca distended by watery or frothy yellow/grey/orange contents. In chronic cases, white casts may be seen (18).
Diagnosis is made by demonstrating large numbers of these motile protozoa in smears made from caecal contents. Samples must be very fresh, since trichomonads are very temperature sensitive, which makes their detection more difficult. Smears should be thin and made in saline. When seen in fresh smears made with saline, *T. phasiani* measures approx. 10×5 mm, moves in a rotational fashion, is circular or pyriform in shape, has a prominent undulating membrane and has an obvious axostyle protruding from the posterior aspect. Several active flagella are visible at the anterior pole although it is difficult to count the actual number, which is four, in fresh material. Giemsa or iodine staining may increase visibility.
ii. Prevention of trichomoniasis has largely been through medication of the feed of growing pheasants with dimetridazole at 125–200 ppm. Nevertheless, outbreaks of trichomoniasis can occur despite feed medication, so then perform treatment with dimetridazole at 40 g per 30 l of drinking water daily for 5 days followed by 20 g per 30 l for a further 9 days.
Dimetridazole for use in gamebirds is likely to become unavailable, so greater attention to management, husbandry, stocking densities, etc., will be necessary to control this important disease.
iii. Several bacterial and protozoal conditions can lead to the formation of caecal casts. Idiopathic caecal cores and mortality have been described in partridges. Infections with *Salmonella binza*, *S. derby*, *S. enteritidis* and *Clostridium cloinum* can result in the condition referred to as ulcerative enteritis or quail disease. Other protozoa that can cause problems in gamebirds are *Eimeria*, *Histomonas meleagridis* and *Hexamita meleagridis*.

19 i. What is the condition and its aetiology (shown in its early stage in **19a** and a more advanced stage in **19b**) in this blue-fronted Amazon parrot (*Amazona aestiva*).
ii. What is the treatment?

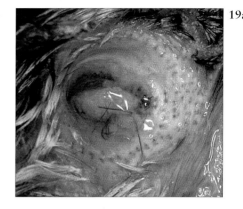

19a

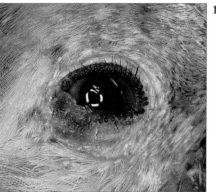

19b

20 During a physical examination on a six-month-old ostrich, the veterinarian has exposed a firm tissue mass (**20**) from the ventral aspect of the cloaca.
i. What is this tissue mass?
ii. Is there any difference between male and female ostriches? Emus? Rheas?
iii. What options are available to determine the sex of monomorphic juvenile ratites?

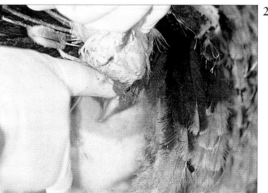

20

19, 20: Answers

19c

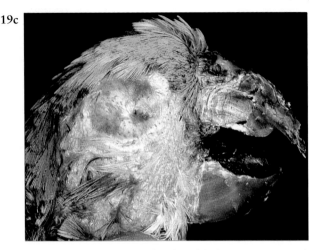

19 i. **19a** is conjunctivitis purulenta and **19b** is blepharitis crustosa, due to poxvirus infection.

ii. Local cutaneous and mucosal forms of avipox infections are the most important viral infections in avian ophthalmology. The disorder progresses more or less rapidly, depending on the virulence of the poxvirus strain and usually affects several birds at the same time. In the early stage, purulent conjunctivitis is diagnosed followed by typical conjunctivitis crustosa. Serious sequelae, which may also be attributable to secondary bacterial eye infection, are ulcerative keratitis and panophthalmitis, as well as severe palpebral lesions with scar retraction and epiphora following damage to the lacrimal and drainage apparatus. Diagnosis includes the demonstration of intracytoplasmic Bollinger inclusion bodies from biopsy material or culturing the virus from the faeces. There is no specific therapy. Administer multivitamins, in particular vitamin A, and provide systemic antibiotic cover to prevent secondary infections. Instil topical antibiotic-containing irrigation solutions and tear replacement fluid. Early removal of cutaneous crusts around the lid is absolutely contraindicated to prevent scar retraction that leads to narrowing of the palpebral fissure, in extreme cases to ankyloblepharon (**19c**).

20 i. The tissue is the phallus of an eight-month-old male ostrich.

ii. The male ostrich chick has a phallus that is conical in cross-section, contains a palpable core of fibroelastic tissue and is characterized by a seminal groove, whereas the hen's clitoris is laterally compressed, soft and lacks a seminal groove. The phallus and clitoris of emus and rheas are considerably smaller and the males are usually distinguished from females by the spiral conformation of the phallus.

iii. Reliable options available to determine the sex of monomorphic juvenile ratites are vent sexing as described above and DNA blood sexing.

21 Bipolar forceps in action (21).
i. What are the advantages of bipolar radiosurgery?
ii. What special considerations occur during the preparation of a potential surgical field if radiosurgery is to be utilised?

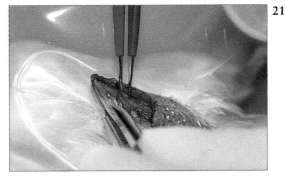

22 This 11-week-old, handfeeding, male Solomon Island eclectus (*Eclectus roratus solomomensis*) (22) has suddenly become a fussy eater, refusing commercial hand-feeding formula (fed at the correct temperature and consistency). Upon physical examination of the oropharynx, this lesion is discovered. A sterile, saline-moistened, cotton-tipped applicator, swabbed over the lesion, is rolled gently on to a slide and is Gram stained. Budding yeast are noted in high numbers. The chick had been treated with nystatin orally, 100 000 U per 400 g body weight b.i.d. for 5 days prior to examination. What should the next step be in the treatment?

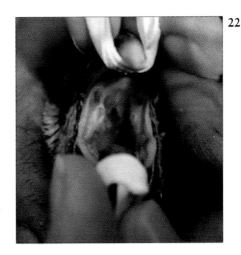

23 i. What is the condition and aetiology shown in this European sparrowhawk (*Accipiter nisus*) which exhibits severe impaired vision (23a)?
ii. Which additional ophthalmological diagnostic procedures would you choose to arrive at a definitive diagnosis?
iii. What is the treatment?

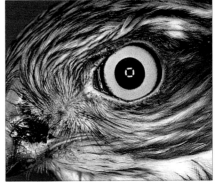

21–23: Answers

21 i. The radiofrequency is focused between the tips of the forceps – this allows a higher concentration of the energy in a smaller area. As a result, it is possible to apply more energy to a desired area with less lateral heat damage to adjacent tissue. This is useful when coagulating small vessels and sealing open capillary beds. This method of coagulating tissue works better in a fluid field than does monopolar coagulation. One technique described utilises the forceps for cutting, however it should be appreciated that the technique is contrary to one of the principles of using the smallest electrode to perform the required function. Therefore there is excessive lateral heat generated.
ii. All combustible solutions can ignite on initiating the current. If alcohol is used in skin preparation it is essential to permit it to evaporate totally prior to radiosurgery. Failure to do this can lead to combustion of the patient.

22 Oral or gastrointestinal candidiasis is most often secondary to some predisposing factor such as prior antibiotic therapy, poor hygiene, some environmental stress (such as being kept at too cool a temperature), malnutrition, vitamin A deficiency, concurrent infection, chemical burns or trauma to the oropharynx from feeding equipment. Efforts should be made to find the underlying cause of the candidiasis.

Nystatin has not led to a response, therefore a change to an azole antifungal preparation is indicated. Nystatin must come into direct contact with the lesions, therefore when gavaged direct into the crop it may bypass the site of the infection. Fluconazole – at 5 mg kg^{-1} p.o. s.i.d. or b.i.d. for 5 days – has proved to be effective. Ketoconazole – at 10–30 mg kg^{-1} p.o. b.i.d. for 21 days – is usually effective although some strains of *Candida* sp. are resistant to ketoconazole. These drugs should be mixed in an acidic liquid, such as orange juice, since absorption will be facilitated and because yeasts grow best in an alkaline environment.

 23b

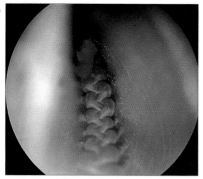

23 i. Post-traumatic epistaxis and subcutaneous haematoma at the supraorbital process.
ii. As 85% of cases of post-traumatic haemorrhage affect only the posterior chamber ophthalmoscopic examination of the ocular fundus is obligatory in trauma patients. The examination is conducted after inducing mydriasis by APA. Induction of mydriasis by the topical application of muscle relaxants, e.g. *d*-tubocurarine, is problematic and carries a number of inherent risks. Of trauma cases, 32% have intravitreal haemorrhage; 80% of the bleeding originates in the pecten oculi (**23b**), a free, pleated projection of choroid into the vitreous body.
iii. Immobilize the patient immediately in a darkened box. Administer systemic corticosteroids. Tissue plasminogen activator (TPA) has been used – 50 mg by intraocular injection at least 24 hours after the cessation of haemorrhage – with encouraging effects in an attempt to reduce the effects of, and increase the speed of, resolution following post-traumatic haemorrhage from the pecten. Euthanasia may be indicated in patients with extensive subretinal choroidal bleeding that leads to blindness resulting from retinal detachment.

24 A three-year-old, pearl white-faced, female cockatiel is presented (24). She is sitting on the bottom of the cage, feathers ruffled and she is obviously depressed. Physical examination shows a bird of good weight (96 g) with a distended lower abdominal region. A mass is palpable within the cloaca; radiographs confirm an egg. What is the currently accepted treatment for dystocia in psittacine birds?

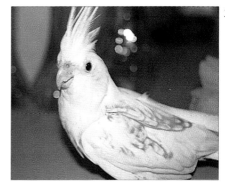

25 The radiograph 25 shows two views, at 90° to each other, of the leg of a 3-year-old female goshawk that was presented lame. The owner was concerned that she might have traumatized the leg whilst out hunting the previous week.
i. What does the radiograph demonstrate?
ii. What is the most likely aetiology of this lesion and how would you confirm the diagnosis?
iii. What is the recommended treatment?
iv. How is the condition likely to have arisen?

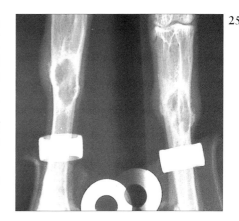

26 What is wrong with the nine-week-old blue and gold macaw chick in 26?

- It is actually normal.
- It is severely stunted.
- It has a splay leg (valgus deformity of the left leg).
- Its defect can be corrected by tying the legs together.

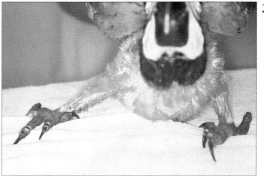

24–26: Answers

24 Initially, dystocias should be managed medically. The hen should be treated with a parenteral multi-vitamin injection and parenteral calcium (0.5–1.0 ml kg^{-1} of 50 mg calcium gluconate and 50 mg calcium lactate per 10 ml drinking water) and should be maintained at 30–33°C (86–91.4°F) and increased humidity. Vitamin D$_3$ facilitates the uptake of calcium. Seed-eating, egg-laying females are often hypocalcaemic and benefit from parenteral calcium. Often dystocic birds are dehydrated. It is extremely important to stabilise the hen and correct any fluid deficits. Any calculated deficit should be replaced over a period of 36–48 hours, 50% being replaced in the first 24 hour period in addition to maitenance fluids of 50 ml kg^{-1} per day. The maximum intravenous bolus for a cockatiel is 2.0 ml. Radiography should be performed to determine the number of eggs present.

Mineral oil per cloaca is not an effective therapy and prevents incubation of the egg. Intracloacal application of prostaglandin E$_2$ vaginal gel is indicated. This gel acts similarly to arginine vasotocin, the hormone responsible for normal uterine contractions and relaxation of the uterovaginal sphincter in birds. Birds do not use an oxytocic system for uterine contractions, so oxytocin should probably not be used in birds. Apply prostaglandin gel directly to the vaginal opening using a sterile, cotton-tipped applicator into the cloaca. Gloves should always be worn by humans handling this drug or treated birds to prevent contact with the skin or mucous membranes, particularly in women. If the prostaglandin does not cause expulsion of the egg within 2 hours surgical intervention is necessary. The egg contents can be aspirated, the egg imploded and removed via the cloaca. A section of the oviduct may be removed to prevent future oviposition.

25 i. The radiograph shows a locular area of bone lysis in the tarsometatarsus.
ii. Such a lesion is most likely to be due to *Mycobacterium avium* osteomyelitis. Biopsy of the mass and staining with Ziehl–Neelsen stain for the presence of acid-fast bacilli is diagnostic. If required the organism may also be cultured.
iii. In view of the poor success rate of treating this infection, together with the zoonotic potential, therapy is not recommended. The bird should be euthanased, and any birds that have been kept in the same aviary or who may have access to ground on which this bird had defecated, should be screened for *M. avium*.
iv. Infection can theoretically arise due to faecal contamination of open-topped aviaries by infected feral birds or following the ingestion of infected quarry or food. In practice, the vast majority of cases arise after the ingestion of infected quarry or food.

26 This macaw has one splay [left] leg, or valgus deformity, which was associated with trauma. This chick had two deformities, a rotational deformity of the femur and a premature closure of the lateral side of the growth plate in the cranial tibiotarsus. This latter defect was corrected by cauterization of the medial side of the growth plate at the age given, followed by derotational osteotomy of the femur 3 weeks later (delayed in order to allow calcification of the femur to occur prior to surgery). If this problem is observed in a chick that is much younger than this one, it can be corrected by hobbling or packing the chick with its legs pushed together in a small container. However, at the age of this chick, the bones are too well calcified for such manipulations to be successful.

27 In young canaries, 2 to 9 months old, an enlarged liver can be seen as a blue spot at the right side of the abdomen caudal to the sternum (27a), referred to by fanciers as 'thick liver disease'.
i. What is your most likely diagnosis?
ii. What can you find at necropsy?
iii. How are you going to confirm the diagnosis?
iv. What should be your therapeutic approach?

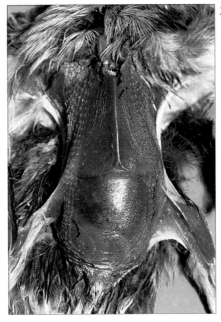

27a

28 A recently purchased five-year old Amazon parrot is presented to you after the weekend with diarrhoea and weakness. A veterinarian from an emergency clinic has given preliminary treatment (doxycycline and multivitamin injections) on the previous Friday night. Despite some improvement during the weekend, the veterinarian decided that further evaluation of the case should be performed by you as the regular veterinarian. During the weekend the bird had shown a marked yellow discoloration of the urate fraction. You decide to perform a Kodak Surecell antigen capture test of a cloacal sample for chlamydiosis and to perform plasma chemistry to evaluate hepatic and renal function. The Kodak Surecell test is negative. The following enzyme activities in the plasma are found (normal ranges are given at the end of each line):

- AST 400 IU l^{-1} (57–194 IU l^{-1}).
- CK 250 IU l^{-1} (45–265 IU l^{-1}).
- Plasma urea concentration 5 mmol l^{-1} (29.9 mg dl^{-1}) [0.9–4.6 mmol l^{-1} (6.0–27.5 mg dl^{-1})].
- Plasma uric acid concentration 300 mmol l^{-1} (5.0 mg dl^{-1}) [72–312 mmol l^{-1} (1.21–5.25 mg dl^{-1})].
- Total protein 55 g l^{-1} (5.5 g dl^{-1}) [33–50 g l^{-1} (3.3–5 g dl^{-1})] with an albumin–globulin ratio of 3.0 g l^{-1} (2.6–7.0 g dl^{-1}).

How would you interpret these values and what further action would you consider?

27, 28: Answers

27b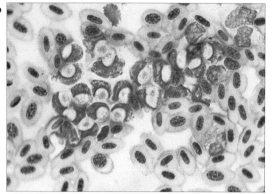

27 i. The most likely diagnosis is atoxoplasmosis, caused by *Isospora serini*, a coccidium with an asexual life cycle in the organs and a sexual cycle in the intestinal mucosa.
ii. At necropsy there is an enlarged, sometimes spotted liver. In the acute phase, a huge, dark red spleen and often an oedematous duodenum with vascularization are seen.
iii. The diagnosis is confirmed with impression smears of the liver, the spleen and the lungs, where the parasites are found in the cytoplasm of the monocytes (27b). The nucleus of the host cell is crescent shaped. Coccidia are seldom found in the faeces.
iv. The therapeutic agent of choice is sulphachlor–pyrazin, 150 mg l⁻¹ drinking water administered until after moulting for 5 days per week, or toltrazurol – Baycox; not available in the USA – 2 mg l⁻¹ for two consecutive days per week. This treatment affects only the production of oocysts but has no effect on the intracellular stages. Additional measures include feeding one part egg food and one part seed mixture to neonates until after moulting. Population control and improved hygiene are recommended. This disease is also a common problem in other captive European finches.

28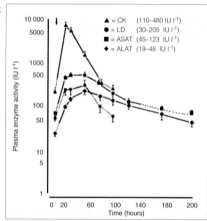

28 The history and response to initial therapy are very suggestive of an infectious disease, possibly chlamydiosis. The yellow discoloration of the urate fraction is probably caused by the multivitamin injection. The results of the Kodak Surecell test from the cloacal swab are misleading since the test was performed three days after the doxycycline injection. The elevated AST is at least partly caused by the i.m. injection with doxycycline. The absence of elevated CK activity three days after the injection can be explained by the relatively short half-life of CK compared to AST (28). Elevated urea concentration with normal uric acid concentrations and elevated total protein are indicative of dehydration with pre-renal azotaemia. The most important action is to initiate fluid therapy. Estimated fluid deficit (10% of body weight) plus maintenance (40 ml kg⁻¹ per 24 hours) plus ongoing losses. One quarter of the calculated daily amount of the first day, slowly i.v. by bolus, the rest can be given s.c. b.i.d. Continuation of doxycycline therapy – Vibramycin i.v., Pfizer, 75 mg kg⁻¹ i.m. once a week for 4 weeks – might be considered since this has shown a good response. Examination of paired serum samples should be recommended and the zoonotic risk discussed with the owner.

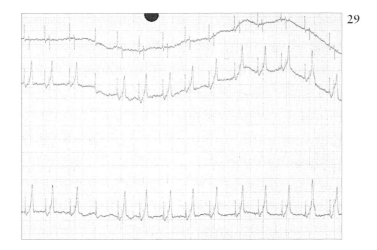

29 Electrocardiography is an indispensable tool for the evaluation of cardiac function in birds. The ECG **29** was made from a racing pigeon brought in for a health check. Standard bipolar and augmented unipolar limb leads were simultaneously recorded with the unanaesthetized bird restrained in an upright position. Needle electrodes were inserted through the skin at the base of the right and left wings and the right and left thighs. The ECG was calibrated to 1 mV cm^{-1} with a paper speed of 25 and 200 mm s^{-1}. What are the values of the electrocardiographic parameters and how should this ECG be interpreted?

30 A toco toucan (*Ramphastos toco*) (**30**) is presented for physical examination. The client has never owned a toucan before but has owned three amazon parrots for three years.
i. What dietary recommendations would you offer and why?
ii. Of which medical conditions – commonly occurring in some species of toucan – should an owner be made aware?

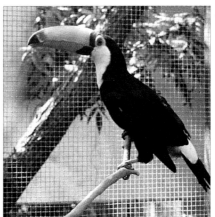

29 The values of the electrocardiographic parameters are (normal range in brackets):

- The frequency is 160 beats per minute (160–300).
- A second degree atrioventricular block Mobitz type 1 – Wenckebach phenomenon – is present.
- The heart axis is -95° (-83° to -93°).
- P-wave 0.6 mV (0.045–0.070 mV), 0.015 s (0.015–0.020 s).
- PR interval 0.065 s (0.045–0.070 s).
- QRS complex 3.2 mV (1.5–2.8 mV), 0.015 s (0.013–0.016 s).
- QT interval 0.065 s (0.060–0.070 s).
- T-wave positive in lead II.

This ECG is normal. The high voltage in combination with the relatively low frequency and the second degree atrioventricular block are interpreted as an adaptation to prolonged training.

30 i. Diet recommendations for toucans contain food elements which are all low in iron. Currently, advised diets are made up of a variety of diced fruits and a free choice availability of dry, kibbled dog food or a commercially available soft bill diet. Recommended poultry dietary iron levels (40–60 ppm) are used as a guideline for ramphastides. It is recommended that a dry ration with an iron level less than 100 ppm is used. Fruit must be offered in bite size portions as ramphastides, unlike psittacines, do not chew or bite their food. Favourite fruits tend to be grapes, melon, papayas and berries. Citrus fruits may enhance the bioavailability and subsequent uptake of dietary iron, so limiting the ascorbic acid-containing fruits in the diet is recommended. Toucans that are rearing young should also be offered live foods such as pinkie mice, mealworms and crickets.

ii. The most significant condition affecting many species of toucans is iron storage disease, i.e. haemochromatosis. Some species are particularly affected (listed below):

Channel-billed toucan (*Ramphastos vitellinus*)
Toco toucan (*Ramphastos toco*)
Keel-billed toucan (*Ramphastos sulfuratus*)
Red-billed toucan (*Ramphastos toucanus*)
Ariel toucan (*Ramphastos vitellinus ariel*)
Choco toucan (*Ramphastos brevis*)
Plate-billed Mt. toucan (*Andigena laminirostris*)
Pale mandible toucanette (*Pteroglossus castanotis*)
Chestnut-eared aracaris (*Pteroglossus castanotis*)
Black-necked aracaris (*Pteroglossus aracari*)
Spot-billed toucanette (*Selenidera maculirostris*)
Saffron toucanette (*Baillonius baillioni*)
Emerald toucanette (*Aulacorhynchus prasinus*)

31 The 18-day-old duck embryo on the left is normal while on the right is an embryo of the same age that was exposed to low levels of insecticide applied to the shell during incubation (31).
i. Describe the pathology exhibited.
ii. With what group of insecticides are these lesions commonly associated?

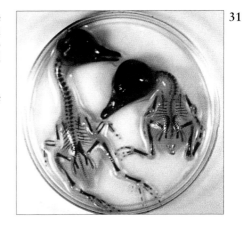

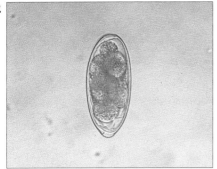

32 Large numbers of the pictured ovum (32) were found in smears made at post-mortem examination from the proventriculus, small intestine and caecum of a pheasant aged eight weeks. However, no adult parasites were found in the digestive tract.
i. What is the name and location of the parasite producing these ova?
ii. Describe the clinical signs that may be seen in birds carrying large numbers of this parasite.
iii. What differential diagnoses should be considered from these clinical signs?
iv. What treatment and control measures can be used?

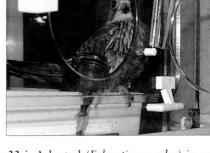

33 i. A kestrel (*Falco tinnunculus*) in an incubator (33) is receiving a form of medication. Explain what this form of therapy is.
ii. In choosing the equipment necessary, what must it be able to achieve?
iii. Which body system is effectively treated in this way?
iv. Why is treatment of this type so useful?
v. Name several drugs that are often administered by this route?
vi. Why can drugs such as gentamicin be safely administered in this way?
vii. As the principal of a hospital using this equipment, is there any factor which could give you cause for concern?

31 i. The abnormal chick shows cervical lordosis, a shortened axial skeleton and subcutaneous emphysema.
ii. These types of deformities are associated with organophosphate insecticides. Other types of malformations include scoliosis, reduction in length of the cervical vertebrae (most pronounced in parathion exposure), incomplete ossification (most common in diazinon exposure) and generalized stunting of embryonic development (also with diazinon exposure). If organophosphate insecticides are required, carbaryl, malathion, permethrin and phosmat are relatively non-embryotoxic if used sparingly.

32 i. This is the ovum of the nematode *Syngamus trachea* – the gapeworm – a common parasite found in the trachea of gamebirds.
ii. Affected birds 'snick', a combination of a sneeze, a cough and a sideways flick of the head. In heavy infestations the birds 'gape', i.e. extend their necks and gasp for breath through their opened beaks. Mortality (especially amongst partridges), loss of weight, weakness, anaemia and reduced egg production may also be seen.
iii. The differential diagnosis should include mycoplasmosis and aspergillosis. Mycoplasmosis is associated with swelling of the infraorbital sinus, between the eye and the nostril and around the eye. In gamebirds with aspergillosis there is usually silent gasping rather than the 'snicking' that occurs in birds with *Syngamus trachea*.
iv. Syngamiasis is most likely to be a problem in gamebirds kept on ground that has carried gamebirds in previous years. The parasite may use a direct life cycle, re-infecting the host species themselves, or use an indirect life-cycle, being taken up by earthworms, slugs and snails, in which they survive from one year to the next. Wild birds also act as reservoirs of infection. Medication licensed and effective against *Syngamus* include anthelmintics of the benzimidazole group and nitroxynil. The benzimidazoles are best administered in the feed, nitroxynil is given in drinking water. Caution must be exercised in using nitroxynil which may result in toxicity, kidney damage and egg production problems; it is not recommended for use in birds over 17 weeks old.

33 i. Nebulization.
ii. The equipment must be able to deliver particles less than 3 μm in size if they are to enter the lung and caudal air sacs. Particles of 3–7 μm generally deposit in the trachea.
iii. The respiratory system is treated by local, topical, application of therapeutic agents.
iv. The air sac system in particular has a poor blood supply, hence parenteral agents may fail to reach MIC in air sac walls.
v. Amphotericin; gentamicin; polymixin; tylosin; amikacin; spectinomycin; chloramphenicol; erythromycin; enrofloxacin.
vi. Amphotericin, gentamicin, polymixin and amikacin are all nephrotoxic. They are generally extremely effective against respiratory pathogens but are not absorbed across the respiratory membrane, and hence they can be used safely without any fear of renal toxicity.
vii. As medication is constantly being pumped into the local environment around your avian patients, there is a potential for chronic low level exposure of your staff to these agents – this is a potential health hazard.

34 Which is correct from the following? This egg (34) is dead in the shell, pipping, early embryonic death or infertile.

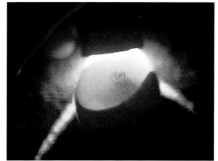

35 Polyfollicular lesion (35) in a lovebird.
i. This is a close-up of the skin between the shoulders of a lovebird. What abnormality is depicted here?
ii. What are some possible treatment alternatives?

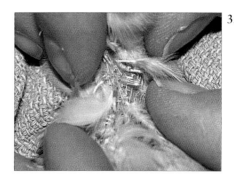

36 High mortality was reported in a pen of adult pheasants commencing egg production, affecting both sexes but especially hens. A consistent post-mortem finding was the presence of grossly swollen, pale kidneys (36) with urates distending the ureters of some birds.
i. What is the most likely cause and how would you confirm the diagnosis?
ii. What methods of treatment and control are currently available?
iii. What other conditions should be considered as possible causes of high mortality in adult laying birds in pens?

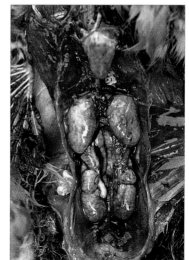

34 An egg that is ready to hatch will look so dense and dark that it often appears dead. Notice the large air cell, indicating draw-down of the air cell immediately prior to hatching. The chick has pipped internally, i.e. broken the chorioallantoic membrane and pushed its head into the air cell. A build up of CO_2 will cause twitching of the hatch muscle which results in pipping. With its head in the air cell, the chick has also started to pip the shell, i.e. external pip.

35 i. There is more than one feather emerging from a single follicle. This condition has been termed polyfolliculitis and is relatively common in lovebirds. They generally present with intense pruritus and self-mutilation. The areas most frequently affected are the axillary and inter-scapular regions. A viral aetiology is suspected but is, as yet, unproven. Isolation of affected birds from other lovebirds is recommended.
ii. The lesions are often secondarily infected, hence systemic antibiotics are usually indicated. Corticosteroid or non-steroidal, anti-inflammatory agents may ease pruritus. A collar may be applied to prevent further self-mutilation until the lesion has healed. However, these measures are only palliative as the condition often reoccurs. The surgical removal of affected follicles may reduce the incidence of reoccurrence.

36 i. Pheasant coronavirus, associated with nephritis and seen in the UK since 1983. The disease most often affects adult pheasants in laying pens. Mortality may reach 50%; white diarrhoea and reduced egg production may occur. Enlarged, pale kidneys with urolithiasis and visceral gout are seen at post-mortem. Histopathology reveals an interstitial nephritis and kidney tubule necrosis with infiltration by mononuclear inflammatory cells.
   It is believed that pheasants become infected early in life; clinical disease is caused by the stress of catching and penning or the mobilization of calcium for eggshell formation by the hen pheasants.
   Diagnosis can be confirmed by serology or virus isolation.
ii. Currently there is no known method of control so treatment can only be of a supportive nature, ensuring easy access to adequate quantities of wholesome drinking water.
iii. High mortality rates in laying pens have also resulted from the viral condition marble spleen disease, bacterial conditions such as *Erysipelothrix rhusiopathiae* and *Pasturella multocida*, septicaemias, predator attacks and poisoning incidents.
   High mortality rates have also been seen in pheasants that have been maliciously poisoned, and in adult pheasants treated with nitroxynil in drinking water to control *Syngamus trachea*. Nitroxynil should never be administered to pheasants over 17 weeks old; also, it can result in kidney failure and death if wrongly administered.

37 i. List the three differing groups of avian ocular shapes, in order of decreasing visual acuity.
ii. Which structure has a supporting role to the ciliary body, thereby permitting a more powerful accommodative function in the eye type (described in i) with the greatest visual acuity?
iii. Which two structures are involved in accommodation within the avian eye? Which one has the greatest influence? With respect to this structure, describe two anatomical factors that enable such a great degree of accommodation.
iv. Describe one main proposed function of the pecten in the avian eye and state why this may lead to increased acuity of vision when compared to mammals.
v. Which retinal feature is present in many avian species, giving such birds three separate visual fields (two lateral monocular and one central binocular).

38 The proventriculus and ventriculus are shown in 38. Through a left lateral coeliotomy, a ventriculotomy or proventriculotomy may be initiated at the location shown.
i. What is the name of this part of the GI tract?
ii. Why is this procedure associated with a higher incidence of incision dehiscence than a gastrotomy in a mammal would be?
iii. What suture pattern is recommended for closure of a proventriculotomy?

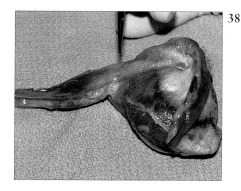

39 An adult, 370 g, blue-fronted Amazon parrot (*Amazona aestiva*) had been housed in a pet shop for several years as the shop pet. It was found dead in its cage the morning that it was presented for necropsy. The bird exhibited no previous signs of illness and no other bird in the store appeared ill. The necropsy of the female bird revealed multiple, raised lesions throughout the liver parenchyma, the lesions varying in size and generally round. No other gross lesions were observed. A contact smear of one of the hepatic lesions was made for cytopathological evaluation (39).
i. What is the cytopathological diagnosis.
ii. How would a definitive diagnosis be obtained?

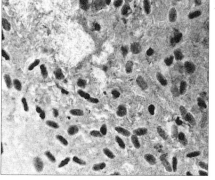

37 i. Tubular, globose and flat.

ii. The scleral ossicles, usually numbering 14 or 15, which encircle the cornea and reinforce the ciliary body.

iii. The cornea changes its shape as a consequence of ciliary body muscular contraction; this has a minor effect. The greatest effect is achieved by the lens: the superior accommodation achieved by the lens arises due to the soft and malleable nature of it. It also possesses an extensive equatorial thickening, an annular pad. When the ciliary musculature contracts, pressure is placed on the annular pad, which in turn brings about extensive changes in the shape of the lens, leading to increased powers of accommodation.

iv. The pecten is considered to be a supplemental nutritional device. It arises from the site of the exit of the optic nerve and may be conical, vaned or pleated. It is thought to supply oxygen and nutrients to the inner surface of the retina. The retina, in turn, does not have any blood vessels in it, which may increase ocular acuity.

v. A unique adaptation of many birds – which enables them to find and catch their food while on the wing – is the presence of three distinct areas within the retina of each eye. These areas are the central, lateral and linear areas, the first two of each possess a fovea. This combination helps in following moving objects. It is considered that in those species in which there are two foveae in each eye, the fields of vision act independently, giving rise to stereoscopic vision, which assists greatly in the estimating of distances.

38 i. The incision is initiated at the isthmus or intermediate zone and from there can be extended orad (towards the mouth) for a proventriculotomy or aborad (away from the mouth) for a ventriculotomy.

ii. There is a higher incidence of incisional dehiscence with these procedures in birds because they lack an omentum to help provide a seal over the incision. Additionally, the wall of the proventriculus is thick and friable making it difficult to invert to obtain a serosal seal. The wall of the ventriculus is muscular or tendinous and generally does not invert.

iii. The preferred pattern for closure of a proventriculotomy is a simple, continuous appositional pattern of an absorbable, monofilament, synthetic suture material oversewn with an inverting pattern to obtain serosa-to-serosa contact. Sutures must be placed and tightened with care to prevent them from tearing through the proventricular wall.

39 i. This oil immersion field is typical of the appearance of this lesion; the smear was stained with Wright's stain. The background of the smear demonstrates numerous bacterial rods that have failed to stain with Wright's. This finding is highly suggestive of a mycobacterial infection because the waxy cell wall of *Mycobacterium* sp. fails to stain with Romanowsky stains. A macrophagic inflammation is also typical of mycobacterial lesions and often macrophages are found full of the rod-shaped bacteria. In this case, a strong presumptive diagnosis of avian mycobacteriosis is made based upon the cytological findings.

ii. A definitive diagnosis for avian mycobacteriosis is obtained by a positive culture for *Mycobacterium* sp., usually *M. avium*.

40 What four factors most affect a fancier's success in the sport with racing pigeons?

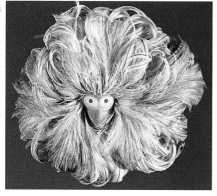 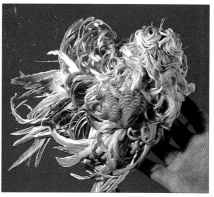

41 What disease are the budgerigars in **41a, b** suffering from? What is the cause of the condition and what advice should be given to the owner?

42 What is the structure and function of the tunnel arrowed in this cranial view of the tarsometatarsus of a typical falconiform bird (peregrine (*Falco peregrinus*)) (**42a**)? What difference is there in this region in Psittaciformes? In distal tarsometatarsal fractures what complications might it cause?

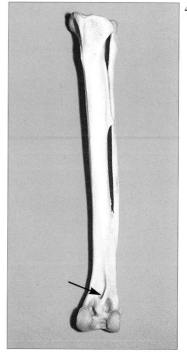

40 The four factors are:
1 Quality of the pigeons – flight performance and disease resistance will both be affected by the individual birds genetic qualities.
2 Quality of the fancier – this comprises various factors, the desire to learn, discuss and reason all aspects relating to health, husbandry and racing of birds. The willingness to invest in new breeding stock, quality food, housing and professional advice is also essential.
3 Quality of the pigeon house and the birds' immediate environment: (1) warm, dry, draughtless environment; these requirements are often neglected. The temperature should be 12–28°C (53.6–82.4°F) day and night. The humidity should be maintained at 50–70%. Air in flow should be above the perching level of the birds. There is a great variation in pigeon house quality and design, the positive and negative points of each house should be assessed and relevant advice given to the fancier. Poor air quality is one of the major causes of respiratory diseases. (2) Environmental changes within the house should be minimized. (3) Excessive numbers of birds per unit area should be avoided. (4) Age groups should be segregated.

41 Birds with this condition are known in the budgerigar fancy as 'feather dusters'; the condition is also sometimes known as 'chrysanthemum disease'. It is inherited and appears to be caused by a single recessive gene. Affected birds show abnormal feathers as soon as they start to feather up and the feathers continue to grow throughout the bird's life. Affected birds usually die at 10–12 weeks of age but on occasions live longer. The grey bird illustrated was nearly 2 years old when the photographs were taken. The owners should be advised not to breed from the parents or siblings of affected birds.

42b

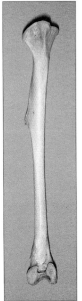

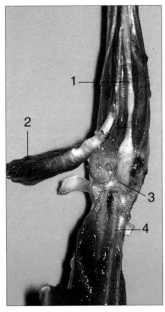

42c

42 The bony tunnel is formed by the supratendinal bridge which runs over the tendon of insertion of the long digital extensor (LDE) muscle and keeps the tendon close to the surface of the bone as it runs over the joint. The supratendinal bridge in parrots, e.g. red-fronted macaw (*Ara rubrogenys*), is fibrous not bony (**42b, c**). If fractures in this region are repaired by immobilization of the intertarsal joint, the tendon's free running will be compromised and this joint, and those of the toes, will be prevented from extending.

1 LDE tendon
2 *M. tibialis oranialis*
3 Supratendinal bridge
4 LDE muscle

43 What anaesthetic systems and gas flow rates should be used for anaesthetizing birds of the following weights with gaseous anaesthetic?
i. 30 g.
ii. 300 g.
iii. 2.5 kg.

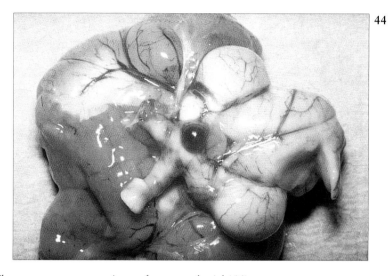

44

44 These are necropsy specimens from a cockatiel (**44**).
i. What is the diagnosis?
ii. What species is most typically affected?
iii. What are the primary clinical signs?

45 Altering the diet of a psittacine is often a frustrating process for many bird owners. **45** is a dropping from a bird fed a normal pelleted diet.
i. How do birds acquire food preferences?
ii. How might the diet of a bird eating seeds be changed to a pelleted food?
iii. How would the nature of the dropping change if the bird refused the new diet?

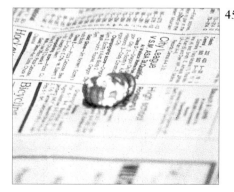

45

43–45: Answers

43 i. Tidal volume for a 30 g bird is 25 ml min^{-1}, airflow required is 75 ml min^{-1}; however, vaporizers are generally not accurate at such a low flow rate, hence use 0.5–0.7 min^{-1}. The use of an endotracheal tube is not generally recommended for birds of this size in view of the small diameter of the tube and the possibility of obstruction with respiratory secretions. However, the placement of an endotracheal tube does facilitate positive pressure ventilation in the event of respiratory arrest.
ii. A 300 g bird has a tidal volume of 250 l min^{-1}, hence requiring an airflow of 0.75 l min^{-1}. If anaesthesia is to be short, the bird has an empty proximal GI tract and it is not a particular anaesthetic risk, then the bird may be induced and maintained on a face mask. Preferably the bird would be intubated as this will allow an apnoea alarm to be used, as well as facilitating positive pressure ventilation if required. A low dead space, low resistance, non-rebreathing system – such as mini-Bethune; Bethune; Ayre's T-piece – may be used.
iii. A 2.5 kg bird has a tidal volume of 770 ml min^{-1}, hence requiring an airflow of 2.3 l min^{-1}; circuits similar to those discussed above are suitable.

44 i. Pituitary gland adenoma.
ii. The lesion has its highest incidence in budgerigars.
iii. There may be polydipsia and polyuria but clinical signs related to CNS dysfunction are not common.

45 i. Most young birds are taught what to eat by association with older birds during feeding. These food preferences are learned and can be changed with persistence.
ii. When birds fail to eat a palatable food, it is not a failure of preference but a failure to recognize the new food as food. When birds are offered a new food in the absence of familiar foods, recognition of the new food as something to eat, if it occurs at all, will occur within 48 hours. Hungry birds will eat the new food even if it is not the preferred food. Each new 48 hour exposure to the new food, with an intervening week of feeding the original preferred food, is a new experience. This means that the chances of the bird recognizing the new food is the same each time it is presented. Repeated exposure to the new food will result in eventual acceptance so long as the food is palatable. On the other hand, the inability of some birds to recognize a new food as food means that prolonged exposure of the bird to the new food, without other food choices, can result in starvation. An efficient way to introduce new foods to birds is to expose the bird to the new food, in the absence of other foods, for periods of 48 hours at a time. This process is repeated with intervening intervals of one week.
iii. The white material in the dropping is urine consisting predominantly of urates. This material does not change in colour nor does it change radically in amount during starvation. In an anorexic dropping the volume of tan faeces decreases and becomes green. As the period of starvation increases, the shades of green darken, eventually becoming black. This is associated with the decreasing volume of the dropping and increasing malaise in the bird. This process should not be allowed to continue for more than 48 hours in any psittacine and for lesser periods in smaller birds.

40

46 i. What special anaesthetic considerations are there in 'prepping' birds prior to surgery?
ii. What special anaesthetic considerations are there during surgery?
iii. What special anaesthetic considerations are there after surgery?

47a 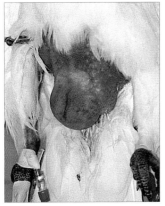 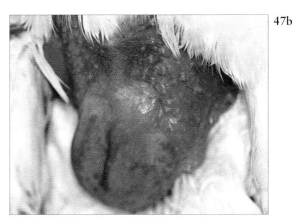 47b

47 This 17-year-old, female, lesser sulphur-crested cockatoo presented with an abdominal swelling (**47a**) which had been getting larger over a period of approximately 2 months. The bird has recently begun straining to void faeces and urine. On physical examination, the translucent skin allows visualization of urates within the cloaca directly below the skin (**47b**).
i. What is the most likely diagnosis in this case?
ii. What therapy is recommended?
iii. What are the two common surgical complications?

48 The lesion on this toucan's beak (**48**) is most likely caused by which of the following?

- Bacterial infection.
- Overgrowth of the beak.
- Fight wounds.
- This is a normal toucan's beak.

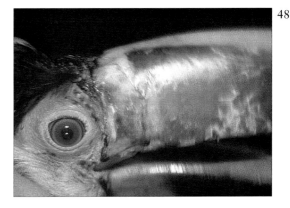

48

46 i. Birds are less capable of maintaining body temperature than mammals, hence hypothermia is a risk. The bacterial loading of normal avian skin is much less than in mammals, hence there is a reduced requirement for extensive cleansing. A minimal area of feathers should be plucked – except in the immediate vicinity of a wound where plucking may result in torn skin – as cut or clipped feathers do not regrow until after the next moult. The use of adhesive plastic drapes helps to reduce the area that requires plucking. Primary or tail feathers should never be plucked, especially not 'pin feathers' (i.e. while still forming 'in the blood') and especially not in flighted birds as damage to the dermal papillae may permanently prevent feather regrowth and hence handicap future flight. Minimize volumes of wash and spirit used. Hypothermia during anaesthesia is a genuine problem so a heated pad should always be placed under a patient whilst anaesthetized. The following table shows heat loss following 30 minutes of anaesthesia.

Anaesthetizing agent	Temperature drop
Halothane	6°C (11°F)
Ketamine	2°C (4°F)
Isoflurane	2°C (4°F)

ii. Body temperature can be monitored during anaesthesia, normal being 40.5–41.6°C (105–107°F). Body temperature should never fall more than 5.5°C (10°F) below normal as this can lead to delayed recovery and circulatory embarrassment. Normal body temperatures should return within 5–15 minutes of recovery. Supplementary heat should be provided both during anaesthesia and until the bird is fully recovered. Recovery excitement is particularly common with ketamine and occasionally with halothane so, as damage may occur to the bird during this period, it should be restrained by being wrapped in a towel or cloth.
iii. Hypoglycaemia can occur post anaesthesia, particularly in smaller birds, i.e. those under 100 g. Such birds should eat within 10 minutes of anaesthetic recovery.

47 i. Abdominal wall hernia. Often the viscera are visible beneath the skin. Palpation or radiography may confirm the diagnosis.
ii. Many abdominal hernias are of little clinical significance. Most abdominal hernias in birds are very large and do not entrap viscera. However, the cloaca may herniate, affecting the bird's ability to void urine and faeces. When this occurs, surgery is recommended. In female birds, the risk of herniating an egg may warrant surgical treatment.
iii. The major risk associated with abdominal herniorrhaphy in birds is respiratory compromise. With chronic hernias, reduction and replacement of the viscera within the coelom can compress the thoracic and abdominal air sac and compromise the bird's ability to breathe. If respiratory compromise is likely, it is better to use a polypropylene mesh to provide support for the abdominal viscera. Caution must be used when placing a mesh subcutaneously in birds as they have very little subcutaneous tissue to support it. Another problem frequently encountered with such herniorrhaphies is failure to accurately identify the body wall. If the border of the body wall hernia is not identified and appropriately closed, herniation is likely to recur.

48 Toucans can be very aggressive to others of the same species with whom they are not familiar. Mate aggression can also be a problem. Hence, toucans should be introduced with great care. Fights can lead to fatalities. Toucans characteristically peck each other on the head, or, as here, bite each other on the beak.

49 This cock pheasant was submitted alive because it was coughing and had a swollen head (**49**). Other pheasants in the pen were similarly affected.
i. What is the most likely diagnosis and how would you confirm it?
ii. What other differential diagnoses should be considered?
iii. What treatment and control measures should be considered?
iv. What is the red plastic structure attached to the beak of the bird? Make appropriate comments.

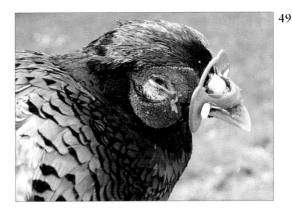

50 One week after a farmer moved a group of four-month-old ostriches to a pasture with long-stemmed grass, several birds showed lethargy, small and firm faecal balls, a distended abdomen and were reluctant to move. One bird had a cloacal prolapse. What is the most likely diagnosis? Give a detailed description of the best technique to treat the affected birds.

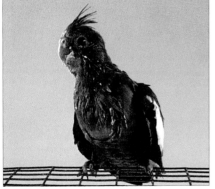

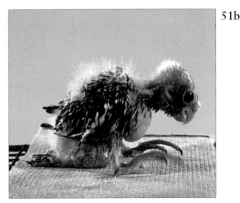

51 The cockatiels in **51a, b** are both four weeks old. What deficiency might account for the differences in their growth and development?

43

49 i. The cock pheasant has sinusitis caused by *Mycoplasma gallisepticum*. The infra-orbital sinus lies between the eye and the nostril and around the eye and becomes distended with mucoid or caseous material as a result of mycoplasma infection. Affected birds may eventually die from starvation or secondary pneumonia, or require culling. Sinusitis has been diagnosed in young birds within the first week of life and in adults; reduced egg numbers and the production of eggs with pale shells can result. The sinusitis is often apparent in the live bird.

Culture and serology for *Mycoplasma gallisepticum* may both give equivocal results.

ii. Other conditions to be considered include syngamiasis (gapeworm), cryptosporidiosis and the following viral infections: Newcastle disease, infectious laryngotracheitis, infectious bronchitis and possibly avian pneumovirus.

iii. Affected flocks may be treated with anti-mycoplasma preparations such as tiamulin, tylosin or enrofloxacin in the drinking water. Severely affected birds frequently require culling. Mycoplasmosis is probably transmitted vertically from adults to chicks via the egg, and horizontally via the respiratory tract, especially at times of stress such as after catching birds from the wild, the onset of lay, etc. Strategic in-feed medication of adults, perhaps after catching or penning or during lay, may help to reduce horizontal or vertical spread.

iv. The red plastic structures pictured are referred to as 'spectacles', employed to reduce pecking of eggs or other birds.

Sinusitis appears to be more common in gamebirds fitted with spectacles.

50 The most likely condition affecting the birds is proventricular impaction with long-stemmed grass. Early diagnosis and surgical intervention are the keys to successful treatment. The caudal and dorsal extremities of an impacted proventriculus can be palpated on the left side of the abdomen. It is important to realize that the proventriculus lies caudal to the ventriculus in the ostrich. A proventriculotomy can be performed after a 15 cm skin incision has been made caudal of the sternum, just to the left of the midline, and the peritoneum has been incised to expose the proventriculus. To minimize contamination of the abdominal cavity, the proventriculus can be temporarily sutured to the abdominal wall before the incision is made. After removal of the offending material, the proventriculus should be closed in two layers with an inverted suture pattern. Antimicrobial prophylaxis is not considered necessary when the surgery is uncomplicated.

51 The differences in these birds are due to different levels of protein in the diet. The bird in **51a** received 20% protein on a dry weight basis and weighs almost three times the weight of the bird in **51b**, which received only 5% protein on a dry matter basis. Protein levels of 5–20% resulted in intermediate growth rates. It is important to note, however, that relatively few nutrient deficiencies demonstrate characteristic signs of deficiency and that the signs of deficiency of a specific nutrient differ among the species. Hence determination of the underlying nutrient deficiency is often impossible. In most cases of nutrient deficiency, in which there is no response to vitamins or trace minerals, it is best to simply replace the suspect diet with one that is known to provide adequate nutrition.

52 Samples from an umbrella crested cockatoo *(Kakatoe alba)* tested strongly positive for psittacosis. A baby cockatiel from the same premises died with post-mortem signs consistent with psittacosis.
i. What is the causative organism of psittacosis?
ii. What test is *definitive* for the disease?
iii. What clinical signs are pathognomonic for psittacosis?

53 During surgical sexing, this lung and air sac (**53**) was observed in a spectacled Amazon parrot *(Amazona a. albifrons)*.
i. What is the diagnosis?
ii. How would you treat this bird?

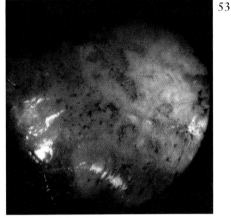

53

54 A pet bird owner calls your clinic because she found her bird chewing on a house plant (**54**). She is worried that it could be poisonous and does not know what to do.
i. What would the proper response be to this owner?
ii. What are the primary problems with inappropriate plant ingestion?
iii. How would you treat the case?

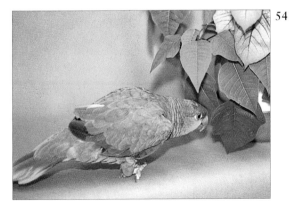

54

45

52–54: Answers

52 i. *Chlamydia psittaci.* Other antigenically related species of chlamydia include *C. trachomatis* and *C. pneumonia* which are restricted to humans. *C. psittaci* has a wide host spectrum among birds including most psittaciformes and at least 130 non-psittaciformes, mammals (horses; cattle; sheep; cats; guinea pigs; dogs) and humans. *C. psittaci* can be highly contagious and induces a disease called psittacosis in parrots and ornithosis in all other animals and man.

ii. Cell culture is the 'gold standard'. Cell culture is sensitive and able to detect small numbers of chlamydia within two or three passages. Unfortunately it is only performed by specialized laboratories and takes about 2 weeks. Chlamydial organisms are often non-viable by the time they reach the laboratory. Chlamydia antigen and serological ELISA tests are commercially available and can be run in-house. False antigen positives may occur due to cross antigen reactions with certain bacteria. False antigen negatives arise due to intermittent shedding of the organism. Serology can be useful in identifying false antigen results, although they may give a negative result in acute cases. PCR is now commercially available in many countries. The test is very sensitive and specific but takes one to two weeks. The prevalence of persistent, probably lifelong, infection within avian populations may require new concepts in control and differentiation between disease and infection.

iii. Clinical signs *can* include conjunctivitis, greenish diarrhoea, sinusitis, airsacculitis, hepatitis and CNS signs including convulsions, tremors and opisthotonus. Haematology may include severe leucocytosis, heterophilia, anaemia, monocytosis (especially in Amazons) and basophilia (especially in conures). Hepatic leakage enzymes such as AST, LDH, CPK and bile acids may be elevated due to hepatocellular damage. No single sign is pathognomonic.

53 i. The black spots on air sacs and lung tissue are anthracosis.

ii. Anthracosis does not have to be treated. It is often observed on routine laparoscopic examination. Note that there are no signs of inflammation in the areas of the black spots.

54 i. The proper response includes:

- Is the bird showing any signs of ill health?
- What type of plant and what part of the plant did the bird chew?

The frequency of clinical toxicosis from plant ingestion is rare. Most parrots just chew or shred the plant rather than ingest it. Any part of the plant may be toxic, e.g. the leaves or fruit.

ii. The primary problems with plant ingestion are oral irritation, regurgitation and diarrhoea. From clinical studies, there are very few plants that are proven toxic to birds but it is wise to look the plant up to check on any potential toxic effects.

iii. Treatment would include:

- Observation but no treatment so long as the bird shows no clinical signs.
- Oral gavaging of an activated charcoal slurry to inhibit absorption of any toxic plant chemicals.
- Supportive therapy, including tube feeding and fluid therapy. The oral mucosa may have suffered local irritation.

55 Profuse, watery diarrhoea (55) was reported in a loft of pigeons. A high proportion of late-bred young birds were affected. In addition to the diarrhoea, a few late-bred young birds exhibited nervous signs such as circling, incoordination, ataxia and torticollis. The adult birds and young racing birds had been vaccinated against paramyxovirus 1 and had been treated for coccidiosis, worms and trichomoniasis. The late-bred young birds had received no vaccination or other medication.
i. What is the most likely cause, and how would you confirm the diagnosis?
ii. Why were the late-bred young birds the only birds to be affected?
iii. What other conditions could result in profuse watery diarrhoea in young birds?

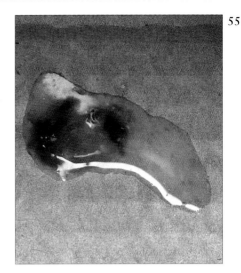

56 A client presents a pet dove for examination. She is concerned that the bird may be a source of 'bugs'. The clinician thoroughly examines the dove and finds it to be apparently healthy and free of obvious ectoparasites. The client points out some creatures on her own head. One is examined under the microscope as shown in 56:
i. What do you tell the client?
ii. How would you treat the dove?
iii. What is the chance of reinfestation?

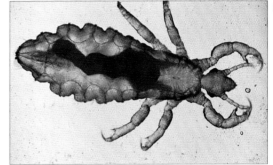

57 i. Can humans infect birds with psittacosis?
ii. What is the incubation period for psittacosis in humans?
iii. What are the clinical signs of psittacosis in humans?
iv. What is the treatment of choice in humans?
v. In which patient types is the disease most serious in humans?

55 i. The most likely cause is paramyxovirus 1 infection which can result in the sudden onset of watery diarrhoea in a high proportion of susceptible birds. As shown in **55**, the faeces consists of a clear pool of urine with a central core of green material originating from the digestive tract. When this becomes mixed by the movement of birds, a 'green diarrhoea' results. Also, affected birds are usually thirsty and a proportion develop a range of nervous signs including torticollis, inability to fly, circling, ataxia and inability to pick up feed. When the birds are stressed the severity of the nervous signs increases. Mortality is usually low except in young birds, but some do not fully recover from the nervous signs and must be culled.

The diagnosis can be confirmed by combinations of:

- Isolating paramyxovirus 1 from tissues such as brain and intestine.
- Demonstrating high antibody titres to paramyxovirus 1 in unvaccinated birds.
- Detecting histological changes consistent with a viral encephalitis and interstitial nephritis.

ii. Although pigeons must now be vaccinated prior to racing or showing, young late-bred pigeons, which are too young to race, may be left unvaccinated with the intention of vaccinating them along with adult birds later in the year. Should the racing teams of pigeons encounter paramyxovirus during transportation or racing, they may bring the organism back into the loft resulting in infection and clinical disease in the in-contact, unvaccinated late-bred birds. An increased incidence of paramyxovirus from August to November has been observed, in the UK, over several years.

iii. Other conditions to be considered include infections with *Salmonella typhimurium*, inclusion body hepatitis associated with a herpesvirus or adenovirus, the motile protozoa *Hexamita columbae* and *Trichomonas gallinae*, and rotavirus and circovirus. Nematodes, cestodes and trematodes may also cause diarrhoea, and chlamydiosis as a cause of diarrhoea in young birds is not uncommon.

56 i. This can be a delicate situation as the specimen examined is the human head louse (*Pediculus humanus* var. *capitis*). Although the dove is not the source of the infestation, it is not appropriate to advise the client as to how to control her own condition. Diplomatically suggest that she should seek advice from her own doctor. A variety of products have been used in humans including lindane and carbaryl.

ii. Treatment of the dove is not necessary as lice are generally species specific.

iii. Reinfestation will not be a problem for the dove. Human health workers can advise her on personal and environmental hygiene.

57 i. Yes.

ii. 4–20 days.

iii. Rapid onset fever, headache, flu-like symptoms, non-productive cough and lymphadenopathy. There are frequently prolonged symptoms or relapses. Pneumonia is seen in 50% of cases as are deranged liver function tests.

iv. Erythromycin.

v. If pregnant or over 45 years old.

58 i. How important is incubation temperature when artificially incubating non-domestic birds' eggs?
ii. What are recommended incubation temperatures for some psittacines and ostriches?

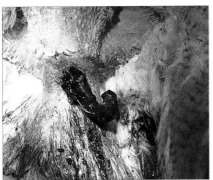 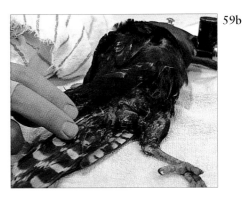

59 Cloacal prolapses are shown in a red-tailed hawk (59a) and a Gabar goshawk (59b).
i. What three structures can prolapse in these species?
ii. What other structure could prolapse in either an ostrich or a goose?
iii. How do you differentiate which structure is prolapsed?
iv. What is the treatment for the three prolapses in i?

60 The two birds (60) are fed different levels of fat in the diet during growth. One was fed 3.75% and the other over 60%.
i. What effects might high levels of fat in the diet have on growing birds?
ii. How might this effect be overcome?

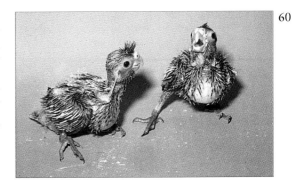

58 i. Correct incubation temperature is critical; the temperature of incubation is particularly critical during the first third of incubation. At this time, a temperature rise of as little as 1°C (1.8°F) can kill an embryo. During incubation, temperature rises of <1°C (1.8°F) for any great length of time can result in a greater than expected number of late-dead embryos. Surviving embryos are often small and weak when hatching and frequently have unretracted yolk sacs. Slight elevations of incubation temperature can also lead to an increased incidence of wry necks, curled toes or scissor bills in embryos surviving to hatch.

Lower than recommended temperatures during artificial incubation can result in late-dead in shell or in weak, often large, soft-bodied chicks due to a larger than normal yolk sac. Even very slight reductions in incubation temperature can delay hatching a day or longer.

During the last third of incubation, negligible changes in temperature (<0.5°C (0.9°F)) have a reduced effect as the embryo acquires some thermoregulatory capabilities and can compensate for slight temperature changes. The only noticeable change may be early or late hatch dates.

ii. Ostrich eggs are incubated at 36.0–36.4°C (96.8–97.5°F), cockatoos and macaws at 36.8–37.0°C (98.2–98.6°F) and galahs and Australian parakeets at 37.0–37.1°C (98.6–98.8°F). As a general rule, small eggs are incubated at 37.0°C (98.6°F) while larger ones are incubated at temperatures ranging from 36.5–36.8°C (97.7–98.2°F).

59 i. Colon, as a consequence of an intersusception (as in the red-tailed hawk), oviduct (as in the Gabar goshawk) and cloaca (which is rare in raptors but relatively common in psittacines).

ii. Male ostriches and geese both have a phallus which can prolapse, e.g. with goose gonorrhoea caused by *Neisseria* sp.

iii. On careful examination in an anaesthetized patient, visual examination will usually allow differentiation, the oviduct being a much larger, fleshier structure.

iv. Cloacal prolapse is treated by a cloacopexi, typically to the caudal sternum or last rib as well as into the laparotomy closure. Both oviduct and colonic prolapse must be treated via a coelotomy, with full retrieval of the affected organ and pexi if the tissues appear healthy. If non-viable tissue is present, either a salpingohysterectomy or intestinal resection, followed by an anastomosis, should be performed.

60 i. High levels of fat in the diet can contribute to the manifestation of deficiencies of other nutrients. Most animals eat to maintain energy balance. That is, they eat enough energy to equal the amount of energy they use. If more energy is eaten, then body weight increases; if less is eaten, then body weight decreases. Since fat is a rich source of energy, high fat diets are consumed at a lower rate than low fat diets. This lower rate of consumption can lead to a lower rate of intake of other essential nutrients. This may result in a deficiency if the diet was marginal in an essential nutrient before the addition of fat. The signs of such nutrient deficiency would vary depending on the specific nutrient deficiency and its severity.

ii. This type of imposed deficiency can be overcome by adding enough of each essential nutrient to compensate for the low consumption of high energy diets. The birds in **60** grew at the same rate in spite of their differences in food intake because each diet was formulated to have the same level of each of the essential nutrients per calorie.

61 Triosseal canal (**61a**). What is the function of the foramen formed by the union of the scapula, coracoid and clavicle? Does it have any clinical significance?

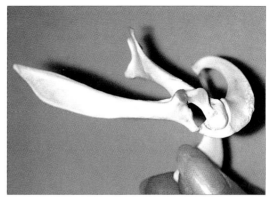
61a

62 If one performs laparoscopy using a left lateral approach from the caudo-lateral thoracic wall, one air sac has to be passed before the viewing field will be as shown (**62**). The picture is of a blue and gold macaw (*Ara a. ararauna*).
i. In which air sac is the tip of the endo-scope at the moment the picture is taken?
ii. Identify the structures 1, 2, 3.
iii. Can any pathological changes be identified?

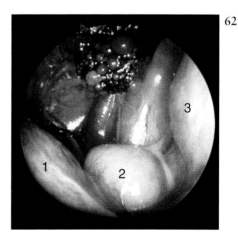
62

63 A keel-billed toucan (*Ramphastos sulfuratus*) is presented for a diagnostic post-purchase examination work up. The diagnostic test performed include a CBC and serum chemistries, a serum bile acid, a total [serum] iron binding capacity (TIBC) and a serum iron level. All tests are within normal limits except the serum iron level. Normal should fall below 6.27 μmol l^{-1} (350 μg dl^{-1}). This bird has a serum iron level of 16.9 μmol l^{-1} (945 μg dl^{-1}) (N ≤350). What is the significance of this value and test?

61b

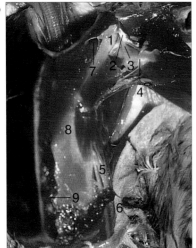

61 The tendon of the supracoracoid muscle runs through the triosseal canal, which acts as a pulley, allowing the wing to be raised by the ventrally placed muscle found underlying the pectoral muscle (61b). The supracoracoid tendon can be ruptured as a result of trauma and the bird is then unable to lift its wing; the tendon must be repaired in order to allow the bird to fly again. Fractures of this region are often seen after a wild bird flies head on into a window. Fractures are sometimes treated by immobilizing the wing though this will allow callous around the triosseal canal to adhere to the supracoracoid tendon causing permanent dysfunction of the wing. Multiple fractures in this region may usually be treated successfully with rest in a restricted area and no immobilization.

1 Coracoid
2 Tendon of supracoid muscle
3 Acrocoracoid ligament
4 Humerus
5 Sternum

6 Ribs
7 Supracoracoid muscle entering triosseal canal
8 Supracoracoid muscle
9 Cut edge of removed pectoral muscle

62 i. The tip of the endoscope is within the abdominal air sac. The visible organs are within the intestinal peritoneal cavity and are clearly visible from the abdominal air sac even though they are covered by the air sac wall and the confluent peritoneum. Introduction of the endoscope in itself causes penetration of the caudal thoracic air sac.
ii. The structures are: 1 – proventriculus; 2 – spleen; 3 – ventriculus.
iii. The spleen can be interpreted as slightly enlarged although this is not an objective diagnosis. The ovaries of blue and gold macaws are melanistic with translucent follicles; all other organs appear normal. Depending on any other clinical signs, a test for chlamydia antigen would be recommended because of the splenic enlargement.

63 There is no significance attributable to an elevated serum iron level in a toucan. There appears to be no significant correlation between the serum iron level, the TIBC, the UIBC and the deposition of iron in the liver of affected toucans. In the past, these values were explored to determine if this would be a non-invasive method for the ante-mortem diagnosis of haemochromatosis in ramphastides. It may be – if a species-specific agent could be developed – that other commonly used parameters such as blood transferrin levels or transferrin saturation values may be useful in the diagnosis of this devastating disease in toucans.
    At present, the only diagnostic modality available in the live bird for diagnosis of haemochromatosis is through a liver biopsy and subsequent determination of iron deposition or quantification of iron present in the tissue.

64 Glucocorticosteroids are thought to provide some advantage in the treatment of head trauma and lead poisoning in avian patients and have been used traditionally for the treatment of avian patients with hypovolaemia, hypotension and severe infection. Unfortunately they have been shown to have profound effects on the immune system of birds and may negatively affect metabolic pathways and organ function. Which of the following glucocorticosteroids would be the best choice to minimize the negative effects on the avian patient?

- Dexamethasone NaPO$_4$ at 0.25 mg kg^{-1} i.m. or hydrocortisone Na succinate at 10 mg kg^{-1} i.v.
- Dexamethasone NaPO$_4$ at 0.25 mg kg^{-1} i.m. or prednisolone Na succinate at 11–25 mg kg^{-1} i.v.
- Prednisolone Na succinate at 11–25 mg kg^{-1} i.v. or hydrocortisone Na succinate at 10 mg kg^{-1} i.v.
- Dexamethasone NaPO$_4$ at 0.25 mg kg^{-1} i.m. or hydrocortisone Na succinate at 10 mg kg^{-1} i.v. or prednisolone Na succinate at 11–25 mg kg^{-1} i.v.

65 A small-scale rearer of pheasant chicks reported that several birds from one group had developed abnormalities on their legs at around five weeks old. This resulted in some birds becoming lame. A typical example is shown in **65a**.

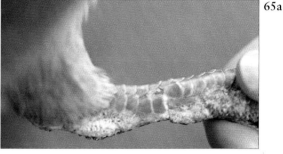
65a

i. What is the condition and from where might the birds have acquired the problem?
ii. How would you confirm the diagnosis?
iii. What treatment could be used on affected birds?

66 This African grey parrot had been chronically ill and losing weight, while passing whole seeds in the stool (**66**).
i. What is the condition?
ii. What is considered to be the cause?
iii. What species are commonly affected?
iv. What tissues should be examined histologically to make a definitive diagnosis?

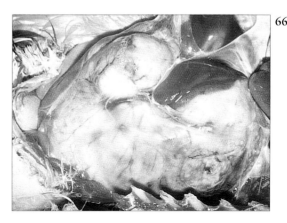
66

64 The correct choice is the third one. The use of ultrashort-acting steroids such as hydrocortisone Na succinate and prednisolone Na succinate will minimize the immunosuppressive and other negative systemic effects on the patient.

65b 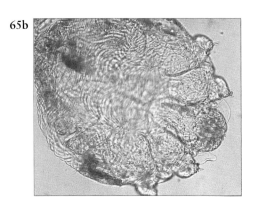 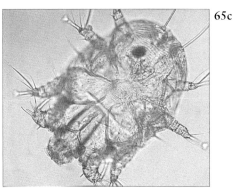 65c

65 i. This is scaly leg, a parasitic condition caused by the burrowing mite *Cnemido-coptes mutans*. Pheasants may acquire the infection if they are reared by the old-fashioned method of using broody hens. An infected broody hen can transmit the mites to her adopted brood. The mites burrow in the skin beneath the scales of the feet and unfeathered areas of the legs. White–grey powdery debris forms on the surface of the scales and between the scales, resulting in the honeycombed crusts visible in **65a**.
ii. The diagnosis can be confirmed by demonstrating *C. mutans* in the crusts. The mites may be visible if the undersides of the scabs are examined microscopically. The adult female mite (**65b**) appears almost round with short legs devoid of suckers. The adult males and larvae are smaller and quite different, having longer legs and suckers on long stalks (**65c**).
iii. Birds should be treated using ivermectin – 0.2 mg kg^{-1} s.i.c. – twice at a 10 day interval; all in-contact birds should be simultaneously treated. Topical application may on occasions be used but is not as consistently efficacious.

66 i. This bird has proventricular dilation syndrome.
ii. This disease is considered to be due to a virus but the exact organism has not yet been confirmed.
iii. Macaws were the first species identified but the condition is seen in many species of psittacine birds. Histological lesions that are similar have rarely been found in non-psittacines such as Canada geese, toucans, spoonbills and finches.
iv. The nerves and nerve ganglia of the proventriculus and ventriculus have the highest incidence of lesion development but histological changes are occasionally found in other portions of the GI tract. Crop biopsy is taken to include a blood vessel – usually including a nerve – in which lesions may be seen. Occasionally, lesions will also be found in peripheral nerves and the CNS.

67 You examine a nine-year-old salmon-crested cockatoo (*Cacatua moluccensis*) that was purchased from a breeder. As part of your health assessment, you perform a haemogram. You note these abnormalities (67) within some erythrocytes.
i. Identify them.
ii. Describe the treatment.
iii. What can you tell the client regarding the origin of the bird?

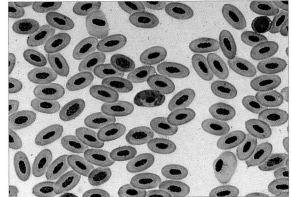

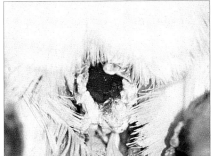

68 This 12-year-old, male umbrella cockatoo presented for tissue protruding from the vent (68).
i. What is the most likely diagnosis for this tissue in this species of bird?
ii. Describe three surgical treatments recommended for this condition.
iii. What is the aetiology and likelihood of recurrence?

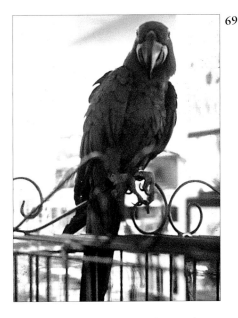

69 This is a hyacinth (or hyacinthine) macaw (69). International trade in this species is restricted due to listing on which of the following?

• Appendix I of CITES.
• Appendix II of CITES.
• US Endangered Species List.
• Brazilian National Protection.

67 i. *Haemoproteus* sp.

ii. This parasite is rarely, if ever, pathogenic in psittacine birds, hence therapy is probably unnecessary, though chloroquine at 250 mg per 120 ml drinking water for 14 days has been successfully used.

iii. The bird was most likely a wild caught import, raising questions as to the bird's supposed history of being captive bred.

68 i. The most likely diagnosis is cloacal prolapse.

ii. Rib cloacopexy, incisional cloacopexy and body wall cloacopexy are the three most commonly used techniques to maintain the cloaca in the reduced position. Because of the high recurrence rate, these procedures are often used in combination. For all cloacopexy techniques it is important to remove the ventral fat pad on the surface of the cloaca as fat will inhibit scar tissue formation, resulting in breakdown of adhesions and recurrence of the prolapse. For the rib cloacopexy a moist, cotton-tipped applicator is inserted into the cloaca to push the cloaca cranially as far as possible. Sutures are placed through the craniolateral extent on each side of the urodeum of the cloaca and around the last rib on each side (usually two sutures are placed on each side). With an incisional cloacopexy, the ventral aspect of the cloaca is sutured into the body wall. A ventral midline incision is made and the fat removed from the ventral aspect of the cloaca. Sutures are passed from one side of the body wall, through the full thickness of the cloaca, and through the other side of the body wall in a simple interrupted pattern, sandwiching the cloaca between the sides of the body wall. The body wall cloacopexy is performed by making two parallel incisions in the serosal surface of the coprodeum on each side of midline. Corresponding incisions are made in the peritoneal surface of the body wall at points that will maintain the cloaca in position, with slight inversion of the vent. Sutures are placed between each side of each incision so that the subserosal tissues are in contact and the serosal surfaces of the cloaca and peritoneum are sutured in two rows on each side of midline. The ventral midline incision is closed and the skin is closed in a separate layer. These are used for definitive treatment. Often a purse string or transvent sutures are used temporarily to prevent recurrence following reduction of the prolapse; however, recurrence following suture removal is common.

iii. The aetiology for cloacal prolapse is unknown. Chronic bacterial infection and chronic hormonal influences have been proposed as potential aetiologies. Recurrence is very common, even following cloacopexy. As a result, many surgeons use a combination of techniques. Castration may be helpful in some cases where it appears that the prolapse is related to chronic masturbation or hormonal influences. Hormone injections may also prove to be beneficial in some cases.

69 International trade in the hyacinth macaw is limited by CITES, an international treaty with over 100 signatory countries. Listing on Appendix I restricts only international trade. Such trade requires an import as well as an export permit. The hyacinth macaw is not listed on the US Endangered Species List.

70 The parrot in the X-ray (70) presented with mild respiratory signs that were exaggerated when stressed for cardiopulmonary evaluation. On auscultation over the left dorsal thoracic region, dull to no air sac sounds were heard.
i. What is the differential diagnosis?
ii. How would you confirm the diagnosis?

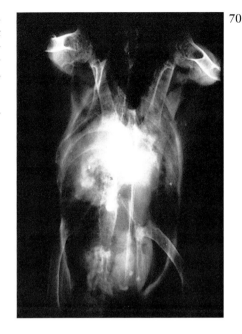

71 These feathers (71) – from a blue and gold macaw – have not been unzipped properly. They are presented for general physical examination. Is the bird well?

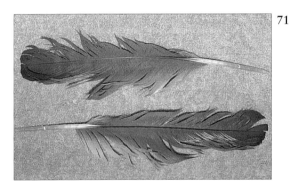

72 Why is it essential to visit a client's pigeon house?

70 i. The differential diagnoses are fungal – aspergilloma – granuloma, abscess of the right lung and abscess of the right cranial air sac. Because of the size and irregularity of the mass, abscess was more probable than granuloma.
ii. Endoscopic examination with culture and sensitivity indicated a large abscess of the lung and air sac involving *E. coli*.

71 i. These feathers reveal that the bird has not been preening normally – the secondary barbs are not lined up properly or attached to each other The process of preening causes the secondary barbs to be attached to each other by the tertiary barbs or 'barbules', which interlock to hold the secondary barbs together in a neat row. The bird may not be feeling well and may be suffering from any one of a great number of ailments. A differential diagnostic list would include any underlying systemic illness, especially those that cause inflammation, including skeletal stiffness or rigidity as a consequence of any traumatic injury, chronic sub-optimal nutrition or emotional stress. The first step is to obtain a data base including CBC, serum chemistry, bacterial culture and sensitivity, and faecal examination. Other tests which may be of value are protein electrophoresis, psittacosis serology, psittacine beak and feather disease DNA probe and radiographs. The depth of testing required for each individual case will be governed by information received or collected during history taking and the physical examination. Environmental factors should be examined, especially with regard to the possibility of exposure to aerosolised irritants, including tobacco smoke. Also important in the history are any factors that may be responsible for emotional stress, such as the loss of a family member, a new baby or pet within the household, divorce, a recent move from one part of the house to another, one home to another or a new cage.

72 Visiting pigeon houses is the only way to assess their husbandry, environmental control, disease prevention measures, stock selection, etc. The observations made during the site inspection should include:

- The location of the facility and the degree of isolation provided.
- The direction the house is facing, a south-east exposure being ideal.
- The type of materials used in the construction.
- The sizes of the pigeon house and the stocking density.
- The area of glass used in the house design (front and roof).
- The slope and height of the roof and the materials used.
- The ventilation system.
- Vegetation, fences or buildings around the house which might reduce the air flow.

During visits, some standard questions should be:

- Which racing system is the fancier using during the racing season?
- How many youngsters will be bred and over what period of time?
- How many pigeons are held per compartment?
- What selection criteria are used at each selection stage?
- What racing success has been achieved in recent years?
- Are recent results improved on those of the past?
- Can any alterations in performance be linked to previous changes in the facility?

Visiting each pigeon house is also a learning procedure for most veterinarians.

73 A seven-year-old female cockatiel is presented with a complaint of diarrhoea. The clinician determined that the client was in fact observing profound polyuria. A blood panel was performed:

Glucose 36.6 mmol l^{-1} (660 g dl^{-1})
Normal range 12.76–24.4 mmol l^{-1} (230–440 g dl^{-1})

i. How would you treat this bird?
ii. What other information would you like to have?

74 An Amazon parrot was presented terminally ill. At necropsy, the liver was markedly abnormal (74).
i. What is the most likely diagnosis?
ii. What are the suggested causes?
iii. Which psittacine species are most commonly affected by this condition?

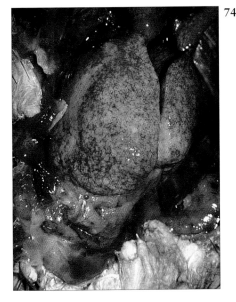
74

75 A young, weaning blue and gold macaw (*Ara ararauna*) (75) is presented by an upset breeder. She had been keeping a dish of seed, including whole, unshelled peanuts, in the weaning cage. She had noticed that the entire peanuts had gone from the cage, shells and all. When she picked up the macaw, she could feel the whole peanuts in the crop and could hear them rattling in the shells. What should you do?

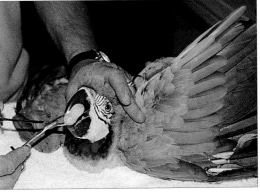
75

73 i. Do not initiate insulin therapy as the glucose level is not high enough to make a diagnosis of diabetes mellitus. Typically, blood glucose levels exceed 55.5 mmol l^{-1} (1000 mg dl^{-1}). Provide supportive measures until the cause of the polyuria is diagnosed.
ii. Investigate other causes of hyperglycaemia including stress secondary to other diseases, hepatic disorders, reproductive activity, steroid therapy, etc.

74 i. Chronic cholangiohepatitis, bile duct proliferation, fibrosis and hepatic lipidosis (cirrhosis).
ii. Chronic infections, bile excreted toxins (particularly aflatoxins), endotoxaemia, and nutritional/metabolic disorders have all been proved or suggested. The cause in many cases may be multifactorial and the exact cause of chronic cases may not be determined.
iii. The highest incidence is in cockatiels, Amazon parrots and macaws, but similar changes are also seen sporadically in other birds.

75 Young birds often present with crop foreign bodies. Feeding tubes are frequently lost in the crop during gavage feeding by breeders, and young birds may eat almost anything. The feeding response in babies is strong, and an object in the mouth, touching the rictal areas of the beak will elicit the response, causing the baby to pump and bob, swallowing just about anything, including whole peanuts.

Many objects, if contained in the crop, can be manually manipulated up the oesophagus and into the oropharynx. The foreign object can then be retrieved with a pair of curved haemostats, as in 75. In most cases, ingluviotomy can be avoided. Most handfeeding, weaning baby parrots can have foreign bodies successfully removed from the crop without anaesthesia or surgical intervention. In order to manipulate a foreign body out, the crop should be virtually empty of feeding formula and the foreign object should be gently manipulated so as not to damage the crop mucosa.

In rare cases, with small foreign bodies such as jewellery, an ingluviotomy may be required. Using isoflurane anaesthesia in an intubated bird, with supplemental heat, a small incision is made over the ingluvies in a non-vascular area. The now visible crop is incised and the foreign body removed. If necessary, warm saline can be instilled in order to cleanse the crop of handfeeding formula so that the foreign body can be seen more easily. The incision should be closed in two layers, initially a continuous simple pattern followed by a Cushing's-type inversion pattern. The skin should be closed separately. If a soft gavage tube is lost, and has passed on from the crop into the proventriculus, it may be retrieved using an endoscope and alligator forceps via an ingluviotomy.

Owners should be instructed to cut up whole items of food and not to feed unshelled peanuts or other nuts to weaning birds. Owners will sometimes phone for advice regarding birds that have ingested whole grapes which can then be felt still intact in the crop. These may be gently squashed between finger and thumb in a conscious bird but the owner should be advised to cut up grapes in the future.

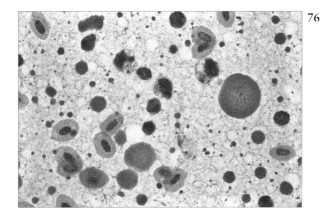

76

76 An approximately six-year-old, female, 38 g budgerigar (*Melopsittacus undulatus*) was presented with a history of laboured breathing. The bird exhibited a gradual onset of lethargy and weakness, with a recent development of dyspnoea. The bird shares a cage with another female budgerigar that appears normal. The birds are fed a seed diet supplemented with fruits and vegetables. The physical examination revealed abdominal enlargement and dyspnoea. Abdominal palpation suggested the presence of fluid in the abdominal cavity. Whole body radiographs revealed a fluid-filled abdomen with loss of detail and cranial displacement of the proventriculus and ventriculus, which contained grit. An abdominocentesis easily produced a yellow, slightly turbid fluid. The specific gravity of the fluid was 1032.
i. What is the cytodiagnostic interpretation of the fluid based upon the Wright's-stained smear (76)?
ii. What is the treatment for this condition?
iii. What is the aetiology of this condition?

77 A young ostrich was presented with severe leg rotation.
i. What are the causes of this condition?
ii. What are the treatment choices?

78 i. What are the indications for using artificial insemination in non-domestic birds?
ii. What are the different artificial insemination techniques used with birds and when is each used?

76 i. The smear is moderately cellular and contains erythrocytes, macrophages and heterophils – the blue granules are either staining or a photographic artefact. The slightly heavy background material contains round vacuoles or droplets, suggestive of lipid material, and small to large basophilic globular material, suggestive of protein aggregates. The cytology is compatible with a mixed cell inflammation as seen with egg-related peritonitis.
ii. Dyspnoeic birds should be provided with a warm, oxygen-rich environment. Abdominocentesis should be performed to remove a sufficient volume of fluid from the abdominal cavity to relieve the dyspnoea. Parenteral fluids, broad-spectrum antibiotics and anti-inflammatory drugs should be provided. Low doses of corticosteroids for 2–3 days will help to reduce the inflammation. Medroxyprogesterone acetate is often indicated to inhibit ovulation. In severe cases, or cases that are unresponsive to medical treatment, it may be necessary to perform a laparotomy and abdominal lavage.
iii. The cause of an egg-related peritonitis can be associated with an ectopic ovulation (i.e. failure of the ovum to enter the infundibulum), a rupture of the oviduct or a salpingitis. The condition may be either non-septic or septic in association with a septic salpingitis or secondary infection.

77 i. Rotational and angular limb deformities are noted in all species of ratite chicks. The causes may be genetic, environmental, being raised on slick surfaces, trauma and nutritional.
ii. Management is the main way to prevent rotational and angular limb deformities in ratite chicks. Weight gains should be linear; only a few days of excess weight gain without proper exercise may induce bone deformities. Proper diet is essential: specific food for the growing ratite is essential to reduce the incidence of leg deformities. A steady growth rate with exercise and proper substrate for adequate footing is recommended for healthy growth.

78 i. Artificial insemination techniques have been developed to overcome the inability of some non-domestic birds to breed naturally because of physical impairment, such as wing or leg injury preventing the male from mounting the female, or behavioural incompatibilities. Occasionally, artificial insemination has been used to increase the genetic variability of valuable birds housed at different locations or because medical management, to reduce the spread of disease, or other problems allow transportation of preserved semen only. The technique has been used for genetic management, especially with endangered species with small founder populations, and for the production of hybrid birds of prey, to maximize various favourable hunting traits found in different species.
ii. Three techniques commonly used to obtain semen samples from non-domestic birds, are co-operation, massage and electro-ejaculation. Co-operative semen donation and insemination was first developed by falconers and involves the use of imprinted birds who have formed close sexual bonds with their handlers and who will voluntarily donate semen. No physical restraint or massage is required as the birds have been properly imprinted. Of all the methods, voluntary donation yields the largest and purest – i.e. least contaminated – sample and hence is potentially the most fertile. The most common method used by aviculturalists is massage. One person restrains the bird whilst massaging its body or legs. A second person massages the abdominal/ cloacal area and collects a semen sample from the male, and then inseminates the female. Electro-ejaculation is primarily used in mammals; however, it has been successfully used with cockatiels, budgerigars and macaws.

79 A cockatiel is rushed in from a flat where the stove caught fire and filled the room with smoke. The bird was immediately evacuated and, at presentation, looked a little stressed, had slightly laboured breathing and occasional sneezes (79a).
i. Does this bird require therapy?
ii. If so, what treatment options would you choose?
iii. What is the prognosis for this bird and can the bird return home as soon as it looks stable?

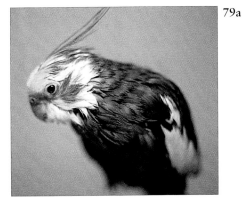

80 i. A wild neighbourhood peacock is presented for the treatment of a leg fracture. Subsequent health assessment includes a faecal flotation. Moderate numbers of ova were visualized.
i. Identify the ovum (80)?
ii. How would you treat this parasite?
iii. How would you prevent this infestation with this parasite?

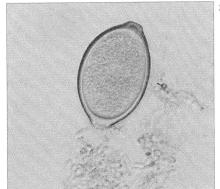

81 i. What is the diagnosis of the lesion involving the proximal dorsal lid of this three-month-old ostrich (81)? How do you obtain a definitive diagnosis from this presentation?
ii. How is this condition transmitted from bird to bird?
iii. What is the treatment of choice for this condition?
iv. Are there any preventive measures to protect birds against this disease? If so, what are they?

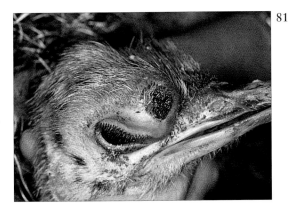

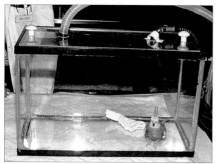

79 i. Yes. Even though the bird does not appear very ill now, clinical disease caused by delayed, complicated pulmonary failure can occur up to three days post exposure.

ii. Treatment includes fresh air, humidified oxygen and, if indicated, bronchodilator therapy, fluids, diuretics and prophylactic antibiosis. Glucocorticosteroid use is controversial in smoke inhalation cases and may be detrimental in many cases.

iii. The initial prognosis must be guarded due to the potential for delayed complicated pulmonary failure from irritant gases released from the fire such as aldehydes, HCl and sulphur dioxide. In view of the potential for delayed reactions, as well as for residual odours in the apartment, it would be prudent to maintain the bird in the hospital for observation and oxygen therapy (79b).

80 i. The ovum is that of *Capillaria* sp.

ii. Treatment of this parasite can be challenging. The parasite often exhibits multiple drug resistance. Fenbendazole (25 mg kg^{-1} p.o. daily for 5 days), mebendazole and ivermectin have been used. Repeat faecal flotations should always be carried out following the discovery of this parasite, to ensure that therapy has been effective.

iii. If the peacock is released back into its habitual environment, reinfection is likely. Periodic testing and reworming is recommended.

81 i. A definitive diagnosis of ostrich pox (cutaneous form) can be made through a histopathological examination of a biopsy sample of one of the lesions. Pox lesions have definitive intracytoplasmic inclusions called Bollinger bodies

ii. The condition can be transmitted through blood-borne trauma, e.g. pecking at necrotic bloody lesions or arthropod vectors, commonly mosquitoes.

iii. The treatment of choice for this condition is divided into management and medical.

- Management – remove unaffected birds from the clinical cases and reduce exposure to arthropod vectors. Affected birds should be cared for in an environmentally stable area with easy access to feed and water. If the birds have trouble drinking or eating, then supportive fluid and nutritional measures must be taken. In most cases, if the birds are managed properly they will survive.
- Medical – since the patients are in a viraemic state and immunosuppressed, antibiotic treatment is recommended, parenterally and topically to the lesions.

iv. Although most avian pox infections are species specific there are fowl pox cutaneous vaccines available. Cutaneous application of the vaccine in the wing web to unaffected birds may provide some protection and can be administered at 10–14 days of age.

82 Which of the following is true about anticoagulant rodenticide toxicity and avian coagulation physiology?

- Birds are more susceptible to anticoagulant rodenticide toxicity than mammals due to a greater dependence on intrinsic clotting pathways.
- Birds are more susceptible to anticoagulant rodenticide toxicity than mammals due to a greater dependence on extrinsic clotting pathways.
- Birds are less susceptible to anticoagulant rodenticide toxicity than mammals due to a greater dependence on intrinsic clotting pathways.
- Birds are less susceptible to anticoagulant rodenticide toxicity than mammals due to a lesser dependence on intrinsic clotting pathways.

83 This female three-year-old Solomon Island eclectus (*Eclectus roratus solomomensis*) is presented with a swelling rostral to the eye (83). The bird is somewhat dyspnoeic, showing upper respiratory signs. The lesion is lanced, curetted and flushed under isoflurane anaesthesia, and then left open to heal by second intention. What should your follow-up treatment regime be?

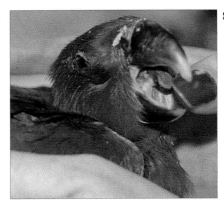

84 A small proportion of budgerigars in a collection show poor plumage and areas of feather loss affecting the body, tail and wings. Affected young birds fail to grow to full adult size (84). Apart from the feather abnormalities and small size the birds appear well and active.

i. What diseases are likely to be involved?
ii. How may these conditions be diagnosed?
iii. What advice should be given to the owner?

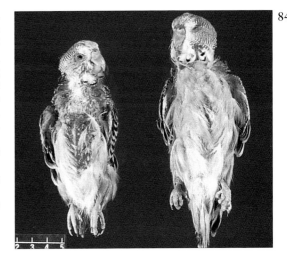

82 First generation (warfarin) and second generation (brodifacoum and bromadoline) anticoagulant rodenticide intoxications, caused by both primary and secondary exposure (in carnivorous birds), are not common presentations in birds even though exposure rates are fairly high. Birds have been shown to be less sensitive to coumarin-type anticoagulants than mammals. This is due to low levels of factor VII and only the minor role played by the intrinsic clotting pathway. Clinical signs include depression, anorexia, feather follicle and subcutaneous haemorrhage, petechial haemorrhages of oral and cloacal mucosa and bleeding from the nares. Treatment involves vitamin K supplementation and, in critical cases, fresh whole blood transfusions. Vitamin K is administered at 0.2–2.2 mg kg^{-1} s.c. or i.m. every 4–8 hours until stable, then the same dose given s.c., i.m. or p.o. daily.

83 Therapy should always be based on cytology and microbiology results. Chlamydia titre was negative. A CBC may prove useful. In this case, a bacterial culture showed a pure growth of *E. coli* sensitive to several commonly used avian antibiotics, including amikacin and enrofloxacin. An acid-fast stain of the debris was negative.

Systemic therapy with enrofloxacin – 7 mg kg^{-1} p.o. b.i.d. – is administered together with sinus flushing with sterile saline (+50 mg amikacin) to mechanically remove any debris from the convoluted avian sinus system. Systemic antibiotics alone may not reach therapeutic levels in the sinuses and nasal cavities in some cases. Fortunately, in this case, response to therapy was excellent and after ten days of therapy the bird appeared normal. Non-responsive cases may require nebulization therapy with sterile saline and antibiotics to effectively treat the condition, or sinus flushing with a combination of saline and antibiotics.

84 i. This is likely to be either PBFD (circovirus infection) or polyomavirus infection (budgerigar fledgeling disease).
ii. The diseases can be diagnosed using blood or feather pulp for the former and a cloacal swab for the latter. The tests are based on the PCR and are available commercially.
iii. Birds showing clinical signs and testing positive for PBFD have the disease, which will persist for the rest of their lives with progressive feather loss. Birds with no lesions but a positive test may be transient carriers and should be retested 90 days later. Polyomavirus-positive birds may have the disease, may develop the disease or remain as infectious carriers for the rest of their lives. Both diseases may also be diagnosed using immunoperoxidase staining.

Unlike the larger psittacines, budgerigars with PBFD do not appear to develop beak and claw lesions. The disease is infectious but appears to spread only slowly in a breeding colony. With larger parrots kept in pairs or small groups it is suggested that the affected and the contact birds are culled – unless they are endangered species – but with the studs of exhibition budgerigars kept communally this would involve the culling of the whole stud.

Psittacine birds should be tested for PBFD and polyomavirus before being introduced into a collection. As the PBFD virus has been found in pigeons and doves perhaps new birds of these species should also be tested to see if they are infected.

Polyomavirus also causes an acute disease of neonatal budgerigars characterized by a high mortality rate which can reach 100%.

85 What is the ophthalmic condition affecting this cockatiel (85)?

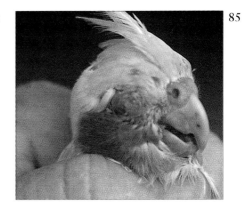
85

- Micro-ophthalmia.
- Congenital atresia of the eyelids.
- Conjunctivitis.
- Eyelids sealed with ocular exudate.

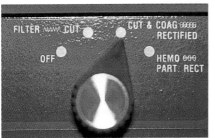
86a

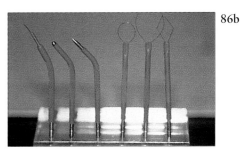
86b

86 During a laparotomy, it is decided that a liver biopsy should be collected. Using radiosurgery to harvest the biopsy, what current and which electrode should be used (86a, b)?

87 High mortality, 30%, occurred in a batch of pheasant chicks from four to 14 days old. 87 shows the typical post-mortem appearance.
i. What is the suspected cause of the problem and how would you confirm it?
ii. What signs are seen in affected batches of pheasants or partridges?
iii. What action should be taken to treat or prevent this problem?

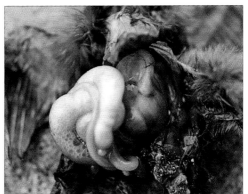
87

85 This is congenital atresia of the eyelids. This is a rare condition and is poorly responsive to surgical correction. No eyelid border is present. Surgical repair is unlikely to be successful as the lids rapidly heal closed. Long-term ophthalmic steroid application may retard redevelopment of the atretic defect; permanent repair is unlikely.

86 The *only* current that should be used for taking a biopsy is the fully rectified current. Because this is the purest waveform, when used with the proper technique, only one or two cell layers are adversely affected creating a suitable biopsy sample. Unfiltered current creates too much lateral heat, resulting in excessive tissue alteration. The advantage of using radiosurgery rather than a scalpel blade or scissors is the improved haemostasis and the ability to reach small, difficult areas within the body cavity. Any size and shape of sample can be harvested with minimal to no bleeding. A small loop or fine-wire electrode should be used. When a biopsy sample is submitted for histological evaluation, the pathologist should be informed that the sample was collected by radiosurgery.

87 i. The caeca are distended with frothy yellow contents and there is evidence of dried diarrhoea at the vent, typical of rotavirus infection. This has been associated with diarrhoea in young pheasants and partridges, young chickens, turkeys, young pigeons and has been confirmed in one clutch of young merlins (*Falco columbarius*).

Group A and group B rotavirus may be involved and can be detected by the examination of caecal contents by electron microscopy or polyacrylamide gel electrophoresis. Group A rotavirus can also be demonstrated by certain agglutination kits but group B rotavirus would be missed.

ii. Mortality, often up to 30%, is typically seen from four to 14 days old, but older birds can also be affected. Depression, heat seeking, diarrhoea and stunting of survivors is often a feature.

iii. Losses in affected batches can be reduced by measures such as the addition of electrolytes to the drinking water and the avoidance of chilling. Antibacterials in the drinking water may help, especially if there is concurrent *Salmonella* sp. infection. If the birds become uneven in size, segregation by size and delaying stressful procedures such as biting and feed changes will help. Measures to stop the rotavirus from spreading to younger batches should be undertaken, including the use of disinfectant foot dips. Regular spraying of birds and inclusion in the drinking water of Virkon disinfectant (Antec) at 1:200 dilution has proved beneficial on occasions.

Many outbreaks are associated with the re-use of brooding accommodation by young birds, exposing them to a heavy challenge by infective particles. If the re-use of brooders is unavoidable, there must be thorough disinfection between batches. Similarly, disease caused by rotavirus is common in large buildings containing several batches of pheasants of differing ages.

Hygiene measures should also include sanitation and disinfection of hatching eggs in case the adult pheasants are excreting rotavirus in their faeces and contaminating the surfaces of their eggs, thus infecting the chicks as they hatch.

88 A Gyr falcon is presented with mild bilateral bumblefoot. Blood screens are carried out yielding the following results:

Fibrinogen: 5.5 g l^{-1}
RBC: 2.8 × 10^{12} l^{-1}
Uric acid: 1021 mmol l^{-1} (17.16 mg dl^{-1})
TP: 48 g l^{-1} (4.8 g dl^{-1})
Glucose: 17.49 mmol l^{-1} (315.1 mg dl^{-1})
Calcium: 2.27 mmol l^{-1} (9.08 mg dl^{-1})

PCV: 61
WBC: 6.5 × 10^{9} l^{-1}
Alk. phos.: 420 IU l^{-1}
Cholesterol: 4.02 mmol l^{-1}
  (155.45 mg dl^{-1})

i. Are there any other details which should be known before interpretation of these results?
ii. Comment on each result, stating whether or not you believe it is normal. Normal (N) values are:

Fibrinogen: <4 g l^{-1}
RBC: 2.85–34 × 10^{12} l^{-1}
Uric acid: <750 mmol l^{-1} (12.61 mg dl^{-1})
TP: 31–39 g l^{-1} (3.1–3.9 g dl^{-1})
Glucose: 13.9–18 mmol l^{-1} (250–324.3 mg dl^{-1})
Calcium: 2.0–2.29 mmol l^{-1} (8.0–9.16 mg dl^{-1})

PCV: 48–55
WBC: 4.2–9.4 × 10^{9} l^{-1}
Alk. phos.: <350 IU l^{-1}
Cholesterol: 2.5–4.02 mmol l^{-1}
  (96.67–155.45 mg dl^{-1})

iii. For any abnormal results give possible explanations of the abnormality.
iv. How would you further investigate the abnormalities?

89 Feather affected by folliculitis (89).
i. How would you describe the lesions seen here?
ii. What infectious agents would you consider in a differential list?

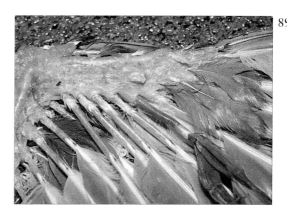
89

90 i. When handrearing chicks, what should the temperature be during these stages: newly hatched; unfeathered; partially feathered; fully feathered; weaned?
ii. What signs are shown by chicks that are too hot and too cold respectively?
iii. Although chicks of differing species will grow at different rates, what general change of body weight should have occurred by day 7?

88 i. It is imperative that the temperature, at which the tests have been run, is known, preferably also the normal ranges for that laboratory. These 'normals' are listed in the question. Also, the time gap between last eating and blood collection is most important in an accurate interpretation of uric acid. In raptors, blood collection for uric acid analysis should be delayed until at least 24 hours after a previous meal. In this case the sample was collected 5 hours after a meal.

ii. and iii. Fibrinogen is raised at 5.5 (N <4); this is an acute phase protein indicating an active inflammatory reaction. Such an increase may well be explained by the bilateral bumblefoot with which the bird presented.

PCV is raised at 61 (N = 48–55); this indicates that the bird is dehydrated. As most raptors acquire all their water requirement from their food, many falconers assume that they do not ever require water to drink. When a bird is ill, on medication, not eating, moulting, egg laying or the weather is particularly hot, they often require additional water.

RBC and WBC are within their normal ranges. The fact that WBC is normal implies that the bumblefoot is either superficial or of short duration.

Uric acid is raised at 1021 (N <750); however, the bird was sampled shortly after eating and is also dehydrated, although dehydration has little effect on uric acid and BUN levels in comparison with mammals, hence this result may not be a valid indication of the uric acid status.

Alk. phos. is raised at 420 (N <350); however, the dehydration and bumblefoot is likely to have caused this.

All other parameters are normal.

iv. The abnormal results may be explained purely by dehydration, timing of sampling and bumblefoot. The bird should be rehydrated over a 24 hour period, then resampled.

89 i. The primary lesion is an exudative folliculitis with secondary feather dystrophy.

ii. PBFD virus (circovirus), polyomavirus (budgerigar fledgeling disease), adenovirus, various bacteria and fungi should be considered, as all can cause similar pathological changes in a follicle. The large amount of exudate and hyperkeratotic debris is suggestive of a bacterial or fungal infection. *Aspergillus* sp. was isolated by culture and easily identified on direct examination in the case illustrated here. The bird also had PBFD, resulting in immune depression predisposing to aspergillosis.

90 i. The temperatures are as follows:

- Newly hatched – 33.3–34.4°C (92–94°F).
- Unfeathered – 32.2–33.3°C (90–92°F).
- Partially feathered – 29.4–32.2°C (85–90°F).
- Fully feathered – 23.9–26.7°C (75–80°F).
- Weaned – 20.0–23.9°C (68–75°F).

ii. Chicks that are too hot will pant and hold their wings away from their bodies. Chicks that are too cold will huddle together, crouch down, shiver and may be slow to feed and empty their crops.

iii. Chicks should be weighed daily before feeding and they should gain weight daily, typically 17% daily in the first week. By day 7 all chicks should have at least doubled their hatch weight.

91 Examination of the faeces of a pigeon with a haemorrhagic enteritis revealed parasitic ova (91a).
i. What type of parasite is likely to be involved in the problem?
ii. What treatment could be recommended?
iii. How might pigeons acquire the parasite?

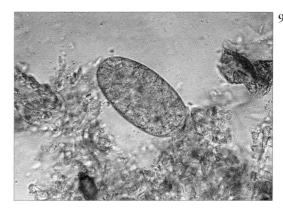

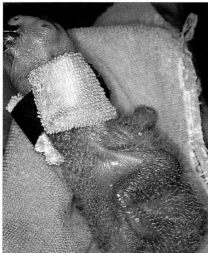

92 The bandage on this African grey parrot chick (92) is which of the following?

• A crop bra used to support the crop in cases of crop stasis.
• A bandage applied to an injury caused by parental abuse.
• A splint used to straighten the neck of a chick that hatched with a crooked neck.
• A restraint device.

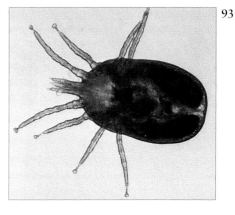

93 A backyard poultry fancier presents a barred rock rooster for a shipping health certificate. During the examination you notice some items moving quickly among the skin and feathers of this fowl. You examine one of these under the microscope and discover this arthropod (93).
i. Identify the species.
ii. How would you treat this problem?
iii. How would you prevent the problem?

91b

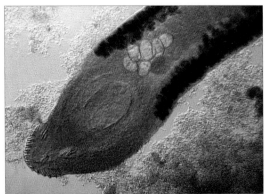

91 i. This is the egg of an intestinal fluke of the genus *Echinostoma* or *Echinoparphium*. The adult flukes measure 3–22 mm and will be detected on post-mortem examination by making smears from the intestinal contents and examining them microscopically. The flukes may also be visible to the naked eye. A characteristic feature of these intestinal flukes is the presence of a 'head collar' of spines and a large, well-developed ventral sucker (**91b**). Intestinal flukes in pigeons have been associated with a haemorrhagic enteritis that may prove fatal.

Although the large eggs are readily visible if direct smears are made from the faeces, the eggs may not be recovered using the standard saturated salt flotation technique because the fluke eggs are heavy and sink. Using saturated zinc sulphate as an alternative to saturated salt helps improve the recovery of the fluke eggs.

ii. Treatment with praziquantel at 12.5 mg p.o. per pigeon is reported to be effective.

iii. The intermediate hosts of these intestinal flukes are snails, small fish and tadpoles; pigeons may acquire fluke burdens by eating snails. Pigeons may be attracted to snails because snail shells offer a source of calcium, needed for eggshell formation. Large numbers of snail shells have been found in the crops of pigeons with intestinal flukes.

92 This chick had a crooked neck which was present at hatching. This is frequently seen and many such deformities can be corrected by the application of a neck brace such as this one. The brace is constructed of a piece of towelling material and fastened with Velcro. The brace can be easily removed for feeding. Such a deformity may be associated with positioning of the chick in the egg or excessive incubation temperatures.

93 i. *Ornithonyssus sylviarum*, the northern poultry (fowl) mite.

ii. Pyrethrin or carbamate powders on birds; spray the environment. Repeat at three week intervals.

iii. Isolate new arrivals: examine and treat before adding new birds to the flock.

94 An adult blue and gold macaw was examined during a routine visit. A blood panel was drawn:

Calcium 4.95 mmol l⁻¹ (19.8 mg dl⁻¹)
Normal range 2.01–2.75 mmol l⁻¹ (8.3–11.0 mg dl⁻¹)

i. What conditions can raise the calcium levels in macaws?
ii. What do you do next?

95 i. What is the condition shown in the eyes of this tawny owl (*Strix aluco*)? **95a** shows the temporal aspect of the conjunctiva and cornea of the right eye and **95b** shows the fundus oculi of the left eye.
ii. What are the differential diagnoses and which procedure would you perform to make the diagnosis?
iii. What is the treatment?

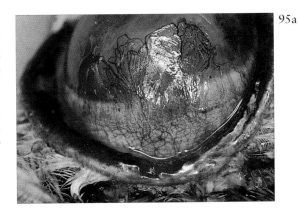

95a

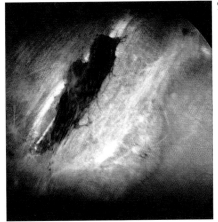

95b

96 i. What percentage of oxygen absorption occurs in the air sacs?
ii. What function do the air sacs serve?
iii. Does the presence of air sacs increase the dead space in the avian respiratory system?
iv. What benefits do the air sacs provide to the avian clinician?

73

94 i. Physiological elevations of calcium occur during the female reproductive cycle. Lipaemia – associated with ovulation or certain pathological conditions – can falsely elevate the blood calcium level. Derangements in mineral metabolism may result in hypercalcaemia. Check for hypervitaminosis D_3.
ii. Determine whether the blood sample was lipaemic. Investigate the reproductive status of the macaw. Review the nutritional programme. Consider radiography.

95c

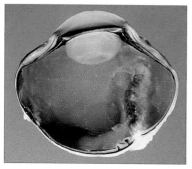

95 i. 95a is superficial and chronic interstitial ulcerative keratitis caused by infection with *Salmonella typhimurium*; 95b is chorioretinitis with marginal hyperpigmentation and severe atrophy of the pecten oculi.
ii. Differential diagnosis in tawny owls includes owl herpesvirus infections as well as other mycotic and bacterial infections, but especially so-called 'eagle owl and tawny owl keratitis'; the aetiology of these conditions remains unclear. Superficial keratitis is characterized by superficial pale red dendritic vessels crossing the corneal limbus. Interstitial keratitis is characterized by the deep blue-red ciliary vessels of the epi- and intrascleral vascular system running dichotomously over the cornea, apparently cut off at the limbus of the cornea. The extent of the corneal ulcer is demonstrated by staining the cornea with fluorescein. The reddening of the palpebral margins is physiological. The anterior chamber – which cannot be examined because of the massive keratitis – is usually found to have anterior uveitis with secondary raised intraocular pressure – secondary glaucoma – attributable to destruction of the pecten oculi: 95c shows the lateral view into a hemisected bulb. The pecten oculi is also important for intraocular pressure regulation. Salmonellosis is diagnosed on serology by demonstrating antibodies, and bacteriologically by examining conjunctival smears and faeces.
iii. The treatment of choice is the administration of systemic and topical antibiotics based on sensitivity testing. Depot tetracyclines are convenient if available and efficacious, e.g. doxycycline 'Vibravenous' (Pfizer). Combined systemic and topical enrofloxacin or ofloxacin is often effective. Chloramphenicol may be indicated in isolated cases to achieve an intraocular effect by penetration of the blood–humour barrier although the side effects and the strongly species-specific half-lives vary widely among different bird species. Supportive local vitamin A-containing eye ointments and tear replacement fluids may be given. Where extensive lesions occur – resulting in extensive or complete loss of vision – euthanasia may be recommended. The prognosis for vision is poor in such cases as shown above.

96 i. None.
ii. The air sacs act purely as bellows, facilitating unilateral airflow through the absorptive surfaces of the lung.
iii. The air sacs lead to a 34% increase in dead space in the avian respiratory system. This can be significant during induction of anaesthesia if using a high concentration of induction anaesthetic.
iv. The air sacs allow visualization of the internal organs by endoscopy as well as air sac cannulation and anaesthesia in the event of tracheal obstruction or surgery.

97 African grey parrot with multiple red feathers (97). What are some possible differentials for the presence of atypical red feathers in this bird?

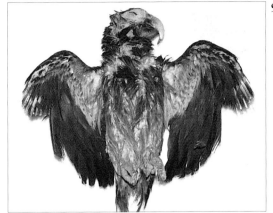

98 This is a microsurgical tissue forceps (98). It has several features making it suitable for use during microsurgery. Describe these features and their importance for microsurgery.

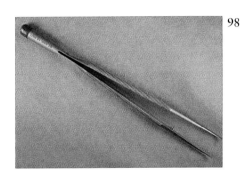

99 i. List the main reasons why isoflurane (99) is a safer avian anaesthetic than halothane.
ii. What are the disadvantages of using isoflurane compared to halothane?
iii. Is the rate of gaseous anaesthetic take up by birds any different to that of cats or dogs? If so, why?

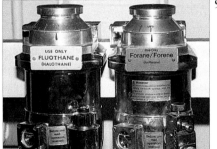

97 Malnutrition – especially deficiencies in certain amino acids – has been implicated as the cause of abnormal feather coloration. Liver disease is commonly blamed for the presence of abnormal red feathers on African grey parrots but it is not well documented. In poultry, hypothyroidism may cause normal black feathers to turn red.

98 The forceps' features are:

- Counterbalance – the back end of the forceps is weighted so the instrument can balance in the groove of the hand created by the thumb and first finger. This allows the surgeon to use the instrument without having to grip it. When the muscles have to hold on to forceps that are not balanced, the muscles eventually fatigue and tremors will arise. Muscle tremors, of course, interfere with accurate tissue handling and suture needle placement.
- Round handles – the handles are round, allowing the surgeon to roll the instrument between the fingers. During microsurgery, the fingers manipulate the instrument with almost no movement originating from the arms and hands. If the handles are flat, the rolling action performed by the fingers is jerky, while if the handles are round, the rolling motion produces a smooth action at the tip.
- Miniaturized tip but standard length – the tips are miniaturized to allow accurate tissue handling of very fine structures during microsurgery; however, the overall length of the instrument is maintained. Many ophthalmic instruments have miniaturized tips but are of an overall short length. Short instruments do not rest comfortably in the hand and must be held between the thumb and first finger. This results in muscle fatigue and tremor.

99 i. The main reasons are:

- Less isoflurane is absorbed into blood, hence induction is quicker.
- Less drug is metabolized by the liver, 0.3% compared to 15% for halothane.
- There are no arrhythmogenic effects, which are well known with halothane.
- Isoflurane causes less respiratory and cardiovascular depression.
- Delay between respiratory and cardiac arrest.
- Halothane in itself is a non-irritant gas and its induction is relatively rapid at 2–5 minutes at 2–3%, however it does sensitize the heart to catecholamines which may induce arrhythmias. Halothane can cause liver disease in chronically exposed hospital staff. Recovery with halothane is generally rapid and uneventful, although it takes a little longer than isoflurane.

ii. It costs considerably more than halothane and requires a separate vaporizer.

iii. Gaseous exchange is stated to be ten times as efficient as in cats and dogs; the avian lung is small in volume and has no alveoli but air moves unidirectionally over the absorptive surface, providing an improved pO_2 gradient and so allowing the bird to absorb a higher percentage of the oxygen from inspired air. The lung is rigid, which facilitates a thinner blood–air barrier, allowing for more rapid transfer. Blood flow is cross current to the airflow direction, improving the efficiency of oxygen transfer.

100 This radiograph (**100**) is a dorsal ventral view of a one-year-old emu showing signs of depression, ataxia, emaciation and anorexia of one month's duration.
i. What is the diagnosis?
ii. What is the treatment and prognosis?

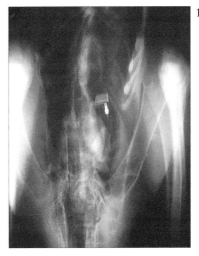

101 These feathers (**101**) show a condition known as achromatosis or failure to lay down normal feather pigments.
i. What is the cause?
ii. What is the significance?
iii. What treatments are needed to return feathers to their normal colour?

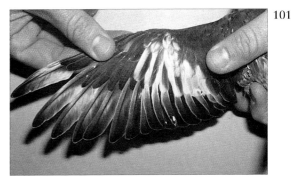

102 i. If you opened a suspected infertile or dead egg, what would **102** tell you about the status of the egg?
ii. What could have caused the condition shown?
iii. What percentage of embryonic mortality occurs during the first and last thirds of incubation respectively.

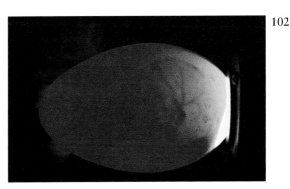

100 i. The diagnosis is a proventricular foreign body, here a cigarette lighter.
ii. The treatment of choice in this situation is a proventriculotomy. The prognosis is dependent on the overall condition of the patient, type of foreign body and if the object has compromised the gastrointestinal tract. Patient evaluation before surgery and supportive care including antibiotic therapy after the object is removed is essential for a successful outcome.

101 i. Achromatosis is caused by a variety of nutritional deficiencies in different species. In this case the cause is choline deficiency during growth. A lysine deficiency during growth causes achromatosis in dark breeds of chickens, turkeys and quail, but not in rock doves or cockatiels. Achromatosis is caused by a riboflavin deficiency in growing cockatiels. In all these cases, birds moult and grow normal feathers some time after the phase of rapid growth is complete.
ii. The major significance of achromatosis is as a serious sign of an underlying nutritional deficiency. Unlike signs of some other deficiencies, it is not dependent on the severity of the deficiency except in extreme cases where the feathers may not grow at all.
iii. The proper course of action is to supply the limiting nutrient and, if the bird is still growing, observe growing feathers for normal pigmentation. When growth is complete, a reduction in nutrient requirements occurs. This reduction in requirements may allow a diet inadequate for growth to serve as an adequate maintenance diet, allowing the bird to produce normal feather colours. In this case no treatment is required.

102 i. The photograph shows a blood ring stage when there is extravasation of blood into a partial or complete ring surrounding the remnants of a dead embryo.
ii. Mortality during early incubation – i.e. the first third of incubation – can result from an improper incubation temperature, genetic abnormality, infection, rough handling or movement, or poor ventilation in the incubator leading to a build up of CO_2.
iii. In both psittacines and domestic fowl eggs, approximately 33% of embryonic mortality occurs during the first third of incubation. The great majority – 60% – of embryonic deaths occur during the last third. The smallest percentage of mortality occurs during the middle third.

103 i. What are the pathological findings in this radiograph (103) and what is their aetiology?
ii. What pathological change causes these radiological findings?

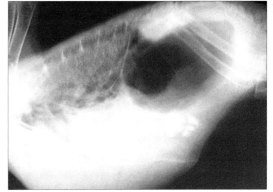

103

104 This three-day-old macaw chick (104) shows one of the following. Which is it?

- Normal abdomen and normal scabbing of the umbilicus.
- Distended abdomen associated with yolk retention and abscessation of the umbilicus.
- Enlarged liver.
- Hepatic haematoma.

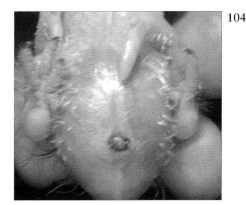

104

105 i. Which bird species is shown in 105? What is the most likely diagnosis?
ii. Which three other organ systems can be affected by this disease in this species. List the organ system which is most commonly affected first.
iii. Which organ system has been reported to be affected in psittacines and raptors in addition to the site found in this species?
iv. How should this disease be prevented and treated. Which problems can be encountered during treatment and how can these be approached?

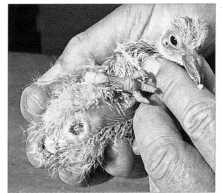

105

103 i. The radiograph shows a distension of the abdominal air sacs, caused by a valve-like obstruction of the upper respiratory tract, impairing the bird's exhalation.
ii. Air trapping is most commonly caused by aspergillous infections. The fungus can occur as plaques or granuloma causing obstructions in the caudal thoracic air sac, syrinx or trachea.

Hypovitaminosis A can lead to hyperkeratosis and hypertrophy of epithelial cells which provoke obstructions of the respiratory airways. Aspiration of small foreign bodies can also cause similar conditions. Tracheal plaques may also occasionally be caused by *Trichomonas* sp. infection.

104 While yolk sac retention is rare in psittacine chicks, this chick has both retention or delayed absorption of yolk material, and abscessation and infection of the umbilicus. The umbilical stump was debrided and repaired and this bird survived aspiration of the yolk material with a syringe.

105 i. This is a pigeon squab with umbilical infection, most likely trichomoniasis.
ii. Upper gastrointestinal tract, liver, heart (endocarditis).
iii. Respiratory system – trachea (bifurcation).
iv. The disease in squabs can be prevented by treatment of the parent birds with a nitroimidazole derivative – ronidazole; carnidazole; dimetridazole; metronidazole – during incubation of the eggs, between days six and 12. However, resistance problems have been reported in the Netherlands, possibly due to subtherapeutic drug dosages given by pigeon fanciers during the racing season. *In vitro* studies have revealed that a fivefold dose of the recommended ronidazole dosage is effective in these cases; experimental pigeons have tolerated a tenfold dose. Other nitroimidazole drugs should not be given in higher dosages than those recommended by the manufacturer. Dimetridazole is well known for its toxic side effects: neurological signs. Overdosing occurs when pigeons drink more medicated water than usual, i.e. when feeding squabs or during warm weather.

106 Treatment for the fracture of the maxillary tip in this Moluccan chick (106) would be one of the following. Which is it?

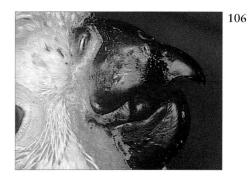

- Glue the tip on with Super Glue.
- Pin the tip back on and secure with a circlage wire.
- Cut the broken tip off as it will re-grow.
- It will heal by itself if left alone.

107 The following abnormalities may be present in chicks at hatching. Describe the possible causes for each abnormality.
i. Early hatch; thin; dry; excessively noisy.
ii. Small chicks or restricted growth.
iii. Sticky or wet chicks.
iv. Unretracted yolk sac.
v. Weak chicks.
vi. Late hatch.

108 Can you explain why birds have a more efficient rate of gas exchange than mammals (108)?

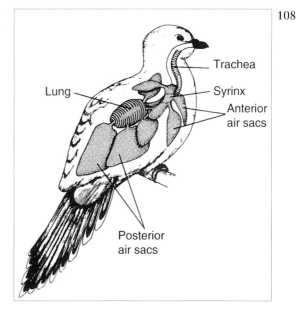

81

106 A fracture, such as in the photograph (**106**), is so severe that successful repair is unlikely. This bird completely broke the tip off before it could be repaired. As the growth centre in the tip of the maxilla was damaged, the tip did not regrow. Less severe fractures can be successfully repaired with pinning and or circlage wires and then strengthened by the application of dental acrylics.

107 i. Excessive incubator temperature; low incubator humidity; high hatchery or brooder temperature.

ii. Small eggs; antibiotic usage in the hen prior to or during egg laying; low humidity during storage or incubation; excessively porous eggshells; excessive incubator temperature.

iii. Low incubation temperature; excessive incubation humidity; insufficient turning.

iv. Excessive incubator temperature; low hatchery temperature; excessive hatchery humidity; yolk sac infection (contracted transovarian, post egg laying as the egg is cooling or during incubation).

v. Infected, dehydrated, cold or overheated chicks; parental malnutrition; incorrect brooder or hatchery humidity.

vi. Low incubator temperature; oversize eggs; overthick eggshell; aged hen; excessive egg storage prior to incubation; infected chick; inbreeding.

108 Avian respiration is more efficient as the lung benefits from unidirectional air flow over its main absorptive surface, the paleopulmonic parabronchi; this is facilitated by the air sacs acting as bellows. With each breath, a bird replaces almost all the air in its lungs, and 50% of its total respiratory system. There is no residual air in the lungs during the ventilation cycle of birds, as there is in mammals, birds transfer more oxygen during each breath. Two respiration cycles are necessary for air to pass through the avian respiratory tract. This allows constant absorption during both expiration and inspiration. The avian pulmonary blood supply is cross current in relation to airflow. These two measures allow a much greater and more efficient oxygen gradient within the absorptive surface, enabling a greater percentage of inspired oxygen to be absorbed. Furthermore, because the avian lung is less mobile than the mammalian lung, being fixed within the dorsal curvature of the thorax, the avian lung is able to have a much thinner blood: air barrier, i.e. the air interface is a shorter distance between air capillary and blood capillary, which facilitates more efficient oxygen absorption. In addition to this, the air exchange surface of the avian lung, related to the volume of the respiratory tissue, is two to four times larger than that of the lung of a mammal of corresponding weight as a result of the very small diameters of the air capillaries.

109 During endoscopic examination of a buzzard these structures are seen (**109**).
i. Identify 1, 2, 3, 4 and 5.
ii. Are there any pathological findings?

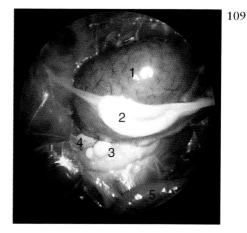

110 What is the significance of and advice on stocking densities – numbers of birds per unit area – in pigeon houses (**110**)?

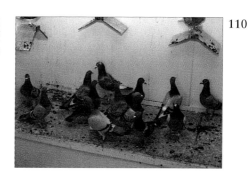

111 This barium contrast radiograph (**111**) is of a female cockatiel with progressive respiratory distress. The bird is eating normally and the abdomen appears thickened but soft on palpation.
i. What radiographic abnormalities are seen and how would you interpret them?
ii. How would you differentiate your diagnosis?
iii. What therapy would you suggest for each of your differentials; what is the prognosis?

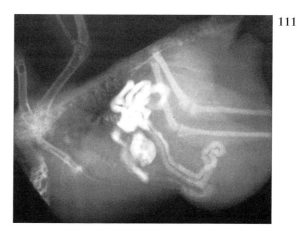

109 i. The structures are: 1 – cranial portion of the left kidney (the colour, size and structure appears normal); 2 – oviduct with the supporting ligament to the infundibulum (this structure is part of the dorsal ligament of the oviduct and is absent in juvenile males); 3 – inactive ovary (note the distance to the oviduct in this bird – if the ovary were not visible because it was covered by intestinal loops, one could easily confuse the infundibulum with a testicle); 4 – adrenal gland, which is always close to the gonad (the triangle comprising kidney, gonad and adrenal should always be identified to avoid confusion); 5 – intestinal loop.
ii. All structures appear normal.

110 Fanciers have a tendency to increase flock size without any increase in the available accommodation. Increased numbers of birds often leads to reduced racing performance. Too many pigeons mean more agitation in the flock, reduced air quality, increased disease incidence, especially respiratory infections. Fanciers should appreciate the qualities of individual birds and be prepared to be selective, either culling or passing on inferior birds. Only the best birds in a loft will make a beneficial breeding or racing contribution to the loft as a whole. Some guidelines:

- Two young pigeons per cubic metre.
- Two females per cubic metre.
- One male per cubic metre.

For young, recently weaned pigeons, some temporary overpopulation is acceptable. This in part is possible because the environmental conditions at that time of year are not so stressful. Overpopulation is highly deleterious during the racing season. As well as the stocking guidelines – which are only guidelines – one should occasionally consider the temperament of individuals or groups of birds. Lower stocking levels may need to be used. By removing inferior birds one can often improve the performance of the better birds.

111 i. The apparent large, soft tissue mass in the caudal abdomen could indicate ovarian cysts, renal neoplasia, a disease of the reproductive tract or ectopic or malformed eggs.
ii. Ultrasound can be used to differentiate fluid-filled cysts, which appear dark – hyperechoic. Abdominal paracentesis may be useful. Removal of fluid rapidly reduces the dyspnoea. Exploratory surgery will provide a definitive diagnosis.
iii. Cystic paracentesis and possible surgical removal will relieve the acute respiratory distress. Testosterone therapy has been used in an attempt to prevent recurrence. Surgery is the only possible therapy for neoplastic disease. In neoplasia of the reproductive tract, surgery may be efficacious. Renal neoplasia is generally untreatable. Removal of ectopic eggs is usually successful although the prognosis is guarded when complicated by peritonitis.

112 An African grey parrot died following a subacute illness characterized by
respiratory signs and elevated SGOT and
creatinine phosphokinase (CPK). At necropsy, the lungs were wet, the spleen was
enlarged and the liver was enlarged and
mottled (**112**).
i. What infectious agents should be
considered in the differential diagnosis?
ii. What histological features can be used
for a definitive diagnosis of each of the
above, and what organs should be submitted?

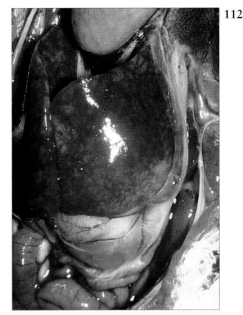

112

113 Propatagium and elastic
membrane. What is the structure (1) in **113**, a dissection of
the ventral aspect of the wing
of a Harris' hawk (*Parabuteo
unicinctus*) and what is its
function? Name the structure
(2). What effect does damage
to this structure have on the
function of the wing and how
should it be repaired?

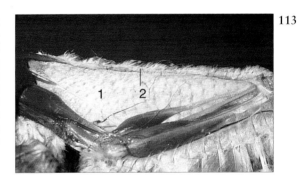

113

114 i. What pre-anaesthetic measures should be taken in birds and how would these
differ between a budgerigar and a peregrine?
ii. State the four most useful methods of anaesthetic monitoring in birds; discuss the
merits of each and state which is the best.

112 i. Severe hepatitis should lead to a consideration of viral infections, such as Pacheco's disease, bacterial infections, chlamydiosis and systemic protozoal infections.
ii. In the liver, the pattern of inflammation/necrosis, occurrence of micro-organisms and inclusion body formation can be used for diagnosis. The spleen and lungs should also be examined as each of the potential causes leads to differential changes in these organs.

113 The triangular fold of skin (1) is the propatagium; it increases the surface area of the wing and forms the aerofoil shape. The leading edge of the propatagium (2) is supported by the tendon of the *m. tensor propatagialis longa*. This muscle has a small, fleshy belly mainly attaching to the clavicle. The distal fifth of the tendon is fibrous and unyielding but the majority of the tendon is elastic and will maintain the tension of the leading edge of the wing even when it is not fully extended, thereby keeping the aerofoil shape while flying; any injury to this area will prevent the bird from flying. When the propatagium is repaired, the elastic tendon must be found and, if damaged, must be repaired by suturing the ends together. Birds can fly well even when they have lost a significant part of the ligament provided it is repaired correctly.

114 i. Pre-anaesthetic evaluation prior to short duration, isoflurane anaesthesia is not usually indicated as the stress involved in collecting samples and carrying out evaluations is greater than the stress of performing the anaesthesia. For longer procedures, the following parameters should be tested: PCV, TP, WBC (+ diff.), clotting time, bile acids, AST, LDH and UA. The crop and proventriculus should be empty. Crop emptying in the budgerigar takes approximately 2–3 hours, in the peregrine it may be 6–8 hours. A bird of prey should not be given casting the day prior to anaesthesia.
    Pre-medication with atropine is not generally indicated. Fluid therapy, given as an i.v. bolus (10–20 ml kg^{-1}) in larger birds, i.m. in birds less than 100 g, prior to anaesthesia and surgery, aids rapid recovery and recommencing eating.
ii. Most surgery requires a plane of anaesthesia in which the pedal and palpebral reflexes are usually lost but the corneal reflex should always be present although slowed in rate. The corneal reflex is the single most useful reflex for monitoring surgical anaesthesia. Automated monitoring is reassuring; cardiac monitoring is most consistently accurate. Recommended respiratory and cardiac rates are given below.

Weight of bird (g)	Cardiac rate (beats min^{-1})	Respiratory rate (cycles min^{-1})
40–100	600–750	55–75
100–200	450–600	30–40
250–400	300–500	15–35
500–1000	180–400	8–25
5000–10 000	60–70	2–20

Heart rate may be monitored by ECG, oesophageal stethoscope or Doppler, respiratory rate by moisture or airflow monitor – apnoea alarm – within the endotracheal tube, or by oesophageal stethoscope. Visual monitoring of respiratory rate, depth and nature is essential.

115 This budgerigar has a bacterial sinusitis (115).
i. What major nutrient deficiency in seeds would contribute to such a sinus infection in birds?
ii. How would you treat the underlying contributory deficiency?

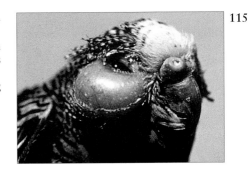

115

116 Birds maintain a high body temperature through endothermia (116).
i. How can they regulate their body temperature?
ii. All birds have a high BMR. Which order of birds has the highest rates of any vertebrate animals?
iii. Flight as a form of locomotion costs more energy per unit time than running. Can you give an estimate of the difference in energy use between a 10 g bird flying a distance of 1 km and a 10 g mouse running the same distance?

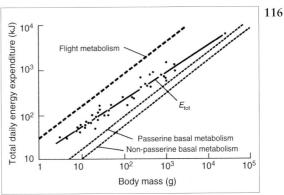

116

117 The extensive corneal ulcer in 117a has been treated medically and unsuccessfully for 4 weeks. What would the best treatment now be?

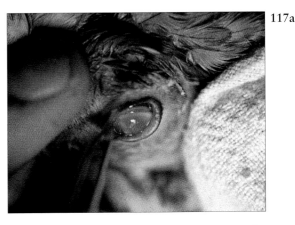

117a

115 i. The specific nutrient deficiency that would contribute to a sinus infection in birds is hypovitaminosis A. Vitamin A deficiency results in the failure of some cells to differentiate normally. In the sinus, the epithelial lining degenerates into squamous metaplasia resulting in a thickening of the mucus that washes the debris from the sinus. This thickening reduces flow rates and allows bacteria and debris to persist on the sinus lining until infection occurs.
ii. Proper treatment consists of antibiotic therapy for the infection and a single dose of 20 000 IU vitamin A per kg body weight i.m., followed by supplementation of the diet with vitamin A. Treatment of the infection without this supplementation renders the bird likely to have a recurrence of the infection.

116 i. Birds regulate their body temperature at 40–42°C (104–107.6°F) by adjusting plumage insulation, increasing heat production through shivering when cold and by evaporating water loss through panting and gular fluttering when hot. In some species, regulation of blood flow through the feet aids heat loss or retention.
ii. Basal metabolism relates directly to mass, although not in a one-to-one relationship. The relationship, in most cases, is given by the formula $BMR = K(W\ kg)^{0.75}$; K is a theoretical constant for kcal required per 24 hours and varies with the species of birds. K is 129 for passerines and 78 for non-passerines.
iii. Although it costs more energy per unit time, flight is generally a more efficient form of locomotion than running. To fly 1 km, a 10 g bird uses less than 1% of the energy that a 10 g mouse would use to run the same distance. The energy expended in powered flight per unit time generally exceeds that of other modes of locomotion, but estimates of flight metabolism are from 2–25 times the BMR with variations that reflect flight mode, flight speeds, wing shape and/or laboratory constraints.

 117b

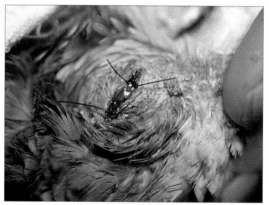

117 A corneal ulcer that is nonresponsive to medical treatment requires surgical intervention. The ulcer should be stained with fluorescein to delineate the margins, which often curl and inhibit healing. After application of a topical ophthalmic anaesthetic, it is necessary to debride the margins and perform a tarsorrhaphy, as in **117b**, to protect the cornea during healing. The tarsorrhaphy should be maintained for 2–4 weeks. Aqueous ophthalmic antibiotic ointment should be applied daily while the lids are sutured together. Partial or complete conjunctival flaps are impossible to perform because of the anatomy of the birds' eyes. Nictitans flaps are of little value because the nictitans is in constant motion and the tissue is friable, which often leads to the sutures pulling through.

118 This macaw had a history of choanal and cloacal papillomas for several years. At necropsy, this is the appearance of the liver (**118**).
i. What is the most likely diagnosis?
ii. What has been suggested as a possible cause?
iii. What other organs should be examined for lesions?

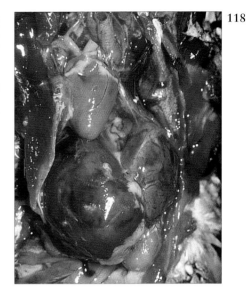

119 A breeding pair of blue and gold macaws (*Ara ararauna*) are laying eggs that are being taken for artificial incubation. Several of the eggs have died near hatch (between 21–24 days of incubation) (**119**) and egg necropsy, combined with microbiology, demonstrates a bacterial infection with *Pseudomonas aeruginosa*. To salvage eggs in the incubator that have not yet died, what would you do?

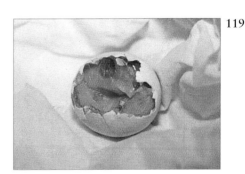

120 This young adult emu has a 'humpback' and crooked neck (**120**). What are the possible causes and treatments for these conditions?

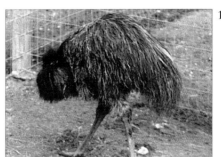

118 i. Bile duct carcinoma.
ii. A virus has been suggested, particularly a possible connection with papillomavirus or herpesvirus but the exact cause has not been conclusively identified.
iii. Papillomas and carcinomas may also be found in the pancreas and throughout the gastrointestinal tract.

119 Injecting the viable eggs with an antibiotic that is effective against the *Pseudomonas* sp. infection may save embryos. A normal, healthy egg should hatch sterile. Occasionally, eggs may be infected by low level bacterial contamination. Infection may occur as a result of ovarian, oviductal or cloacal infection. Contamination is by minute cracks or pin-holes in the shell at the time of handling or egg collection. All eggs should be candled so that any non-viable eggs may be removed from the incubator prior to possible contamination of healthy eggs. The incubator should be sanitized. Piperacillin has been used to treat infected eggs. A small hole is drilled, using a sterile 27 gauge needle over the air cell, and the antibiotic is injected into the air cell. The hole is sealed with white, water-soluble glue (being careful not to cover additional areas of the shell as this would reduce water loss from the egg during incubation). Injections are given on days 14, 18 and 22. The dose for piperacillin is 0.2 ml of a 200 mg ml^{-1} solution. Any chick that hatches should be cultured for bacteria immediately upon breaking open the shell, and antibiotic therapy should be commenced depending on the culture results. Nystatin should be given concurrently at 100 000 U per 400 g of body weight to prevent secondary infections with *Candida* sp. Any chick hatching from an egg such as this will also benefit from the administration of probiotics.

120 Spinal abnormalities have become a common occurrence with farm-raised emus. There are five differential diagnostic categories that may be singularly or multiply involved with this presentation.

- Trauma – many cases of this presentation are related to trauma involving the cervical vertebral area thereby causing abnormal development of the neck during the fast rate of growth. Fast action by the veterinarian using corticosteroids, muscle relaxants and physiotherapy has helped some cases.
- Parasites – there have been parasite infections identified with this presentation. *Chandlerella quiscali* , in particular, has caused young emus – less than one year old – to develop cervical malformations. The parasite is transmitted by *Culicoides* sp. during warm months of the year. Since older birds – greater than one-year-old – do not seem affected, preventive measures are reserved for younger animals. Recommended preventive measures include ivermectin, subcutaneously, i.m. or p.o. at 200 mg kg^{-1} once a month until the bird is eight months old.
- Nutrition – poor quality feeds, vitamin E/selenium deficiencies or Ca/P imbalances could cause the problem. With the advent of easily accessible ratite feed this can easily be ruled out as a cause. It must be remembered that each ratite species has different nutritional requirements and species-specific ratite feed is recommended. Specific toxicities should be ruled out with a thorough history, veterinary investigation and examination.
- Genetics – there is always a possibility of related animals producing chicks with a predisposition to this problem.
- Infectious – bacterial or viral encephalitis and/or meningitis is another possibility. Routine avian work-ups should help rule out this potential problem.

121 This is a solitary pet, a wild-caught African grey parrot purchased one month previously. It demonstrates progressive anorexia, emaciation, polydipsia and polyuria. Tremor and opisthotonus have been observed for the previous two days.
i. What abnormalities are seen in the radiograph (121)?
ii. What diseases are suspected?
iii. What is the prognosis?

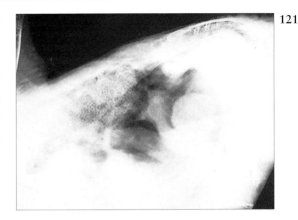

122 A goose was found weak on the shore of a local pond where oil had been dumped. The goose was covered in oil, dehydrated and weak although it was alert and responsive (122).
i. What are the primary concerns with oil toxicosis?
ii. How would you treat this goose?

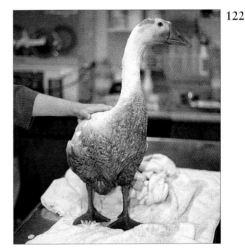

123 i. Why is it important to periodically weigh incubating eggs (123)?
ii. What weight changes are expected from laying to hatching?
iii. What corrective measures can be taken if egg weight is abnormal?

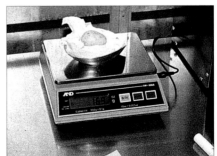

121 i. There are increased densities, notably in the syringeal area and of the greater vessels of the heart. There is a focal density in the abdominal air sac and the proventriculus is enlarged. The bird has a severe splenomegaly as well as renal radiodensities.
ii. Chlamydiosis should be suspected in all birds with splenomegaly. The focal densities in the syringeal and air sac areas may be indicative of aspergillosis. Renal radiodensities are consistent with uric acid crystal deposition. The radiodensities of the great heart vessels may be consistent with uric acid deposition in the pericardium or in the vessel walls, i.e. gout.
iii. The prognosis is poor to grave: there are three potentially life-threatening diseases to consider. Each may involve prolonged treatment and carry a grave prognosis. Treatment of the chlamydiosis may exacerbate the fungal infection. Treatment of the gout may be prolonged and of equivocal efficacy. Continued treatment of this bird may not be justified.

122 i. Concerns of oil toxicosis are:

• Destruction of waterproofing and the insulatory properties of the plumage.
• Diarrhoea arising due to GI irritation following the ingestion of oil during preening.
• Haemolytic anaemia
• Hypothermia
• Pneumonia – bacterial or fungal – due to immune suppression or inhalation of oil.

ii. Treatment includes heat, supportive care, activated charcoal – to inhibit the absorption of ingested oil – and, once stabilized, frequent high pressure (preferably 90 psi/620 kNm^{-2}), warm (40–45°C/104–113°F) mild detergent baths and clean warm water rinses until the water coming off the feathers 'beads' freely. The birds are then placed in a flow of warm air until dry. It is normal to maintain birds in captivity on self-skimming ponds for several days after washing to ensure that waterproofing is secure.

123 i. The developing embryo's metabolism combined with evaporation will result in egg weight loss due to water loss, during the incubation process. This is true of eggs under both natural, i.e. parental, and artificial incubation. Weighing eggs periodically and charting weight loss is an important technique used in monitoring the development and health of an embryo.
ii. Acceptable weight loss from the start of incubation to piping is 13%, and 16% by the time of hatching; however, there is a range of 11–16%. Weight loss is not constant, the greater losses occur during early and late incubation. Charting weight loss is helpful to determine if the egg weight is on target for the time of elapsed incubation. The size of the air cell increases in proportion to the weight loss.
iii. Weight loss greater than expected may be an indication of low humidity levels in the incubator. To increase humidity, place a tray of water, or mist the environment, in the incubator. If further control is required, a non-toxic white glue may be placed on part of the eggshell over the air cell, thereby reducing the area from which water vapour may be lost. As once applied, such glue is difficult to remove, only a small application should be made. Reduced weight loss may result when an egg is incubated at too high a humidity level; it may also indicate an abnormal or dead embryo. Inadequate weight loss can be increased by desiccating the incubator, i.e. reducing the humidity using silica gel. If necessary, emery paper may be used to gently sand the eggshell over the air cell, or a small hole may be made in the shell over the air cell – without rupturing the membrane – in order to permit increased water loss. The egg should be candled for viability.

124 Canary with abnormal plumage (**124**).
i. What is the lesion in this canary?
ii. What causes it?
iii. How can it be treated?

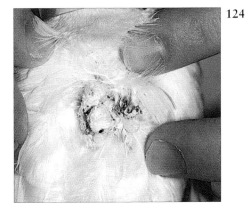

125 A red-tailed hawk, found injured on the road, is presented with dyspnoea. Radiographs (**125**) indicate lesions consistent with aspergillosis; an aspergillus titre is positive. What is the treatment of choice?

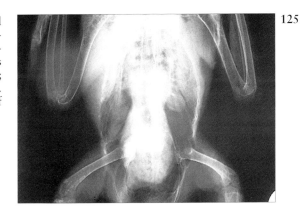

126 An African grey parrot was presented following collapse and convulsions. Its serum calcium was 1.05 mmol l^{-1} (4.2 mg dl^{-1}). The lesion (**126**) was found at necropsy.
i. What is your diagnosis?
ii. What are the potential causes of this lesion?
iii. What other tissues should be examined for lesions?

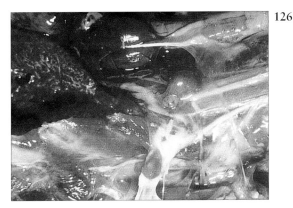

124 i. These are feather cysts. In this example, the cysts involve only body feathers but in some birds they may occur in flight feathers. The lesion consists of a grossly swollen follicle containing a balled-up, ingrown feather that has curled around and not emerged. They often have large amounts of keratin debris in the follicle of the feather.

ii. Cysts occurring in the body feathers of canaries often have a familial pattern and are thought to be inherited although this is not well documented. They may occur secondary to traumatic or infectious damage. Cysts occurring in the flight feathers of other birds – especially cockatiels – are usually the result of traumatic damage to the follicle.

iii. Usually, the follicle must be removed surgically to prevent recurrence. Often, in the case of canaries, there are multiple cysts occurring in a single feather tract. In severe cases, the whole affected feather tract may need to be removed. In the case of a single cyst of a flight feather, the affected follicle may be carefully incised and the feather and debris removed; the follicle is left to heal by second intention. Often, this treatment results in the reoccurrence of the cyst, in which case the whole follicle must be removed.

125 Itraconazole shows the most activity against aspergillosis, in comparison with other members of the azole group. For systemic therapy, itraconazole is less toxic than amphoteracin. Amphoteracin can only be given by intravenous, intratracheal routes, nebulization or direct application via catheters on to air sac lesions. Despite the potential renal toxicity of amphoteracin, in view of its efficacy it is recommended for intravenous use – 1.5 mg kg^{-1} t.i.d. i.v. – for the first 3 days of therapy and thereafter by direct lesion application. Care should be taken to avoid administering amphoteracin to a dehydrated bird since this can cause severe renal damage. Additional i.v. fluid may be given with i.v. amphoteracin in order to minimize this risk. Itraconazole need not be acidified prior to administration in carnivorous birds. Itraconazole should be administered at 10 mg kg^{-1} p.o. b.i.d. with food for 30–60 days. It should be remembered that azole group antifungals are fungistatic. *Aspergillus* granulomas may need to be removed surgically. The bird should also be treated with nebulization with clotrimaziole dissolved in polyethylene glycol (PEG 300), 10 mg ml^{-1} t.i.d. for 20–30 minutes for 30–45 days.

126 i. Parathyroid gland hyperplasia or possible adenoma formation.

ii. Causes include nutritional secondary hyperplasia, parathyroid neoplasia and idiopathic hyperplasia, as well as primary renal disease. The condition is more common in African grey parrots than in other psittacines.

iii. Bone should be examined as there can be calcium loss and osteomalacia/osteo-dystrophy. The kidney and proventriculus should be examined for primary or secondary renal diseases and for soft tissue mineralization.

127 This injury (127a) to the maxilla resulted when the macaw flew into a ceiling fan. Describe the technique used to repair it using dental acrylics.

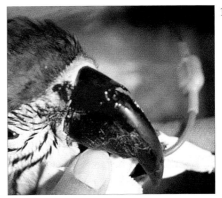

127a

128 An eight-week-old cockatoo (128) presented as an emergency because the owner noticed food coming from the throat. The bird is still being syringe fed and weaning has not yet been started. The bird is bright, alert and active on presentation.
i. What is your diagnosis?
ii. What is the most likely aetiology for this condition given the history and physical findings?
iii. How should this condition be managed surgically and what is the long-term prognosis?

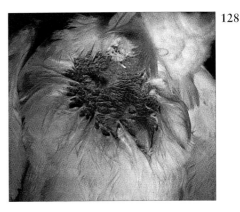

128

129 An adult African grey parrot (*Psittacus erithacus*) was presented with a history of weight loss and periodic coughing. The CBC and blood biochemistry profile was unremarkable except for a slight anaemia where PCV = 32% (N = 35–55%) and slightly elevated TP at 57 g l^{-1} (5.7 g dl^{-1}) [N = 35–55 g l^{-1} (3.5–5.5 g dl^{-1})]. A tracheal wash was performed for cytological evaluation of the upper airway. What is the cytodiagnosis based upon the Wright's-stained concentrated tracheal wash sample (129)?

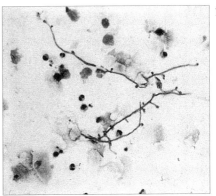

129

127b

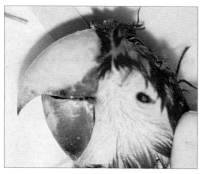

127 A functional and aesthetic repair should be the goal for any beak defect. It is therefore necessary to use a bonding agent that can match the natural colour of the beak being repaired. Most repairs require tones of yellow or black, however in some birds reds, greens, oranges and blues are necessary. Preparation of the beak requires the removal of any loose particles of the ramphotheca and etching or scoring the margins of the wound. The beak should be wiped clean and allowed to dry. When matching colours, very small amounts of colour powder are mixed homogeneously with the acrylic powder to develop the desired colour. This mixture is then mixed with one or two drops of the liquid and quickly applied to the defect. The margin of the bonding mixture should be feathered beyond the edge of the injury. After the acrylic has hardened, over 1–2 minutes, the applied bonding agent should be sanded smooth so that the margin of the defect is not visible (127b).

128 i. This bird has a crop fistula, which is characterized by a fistula between the ingluvies (crop) and the skin allowing ingested food to pass out of the ingluvies.
ii. The fistula is most likely the result of feeding inappropriately heated food to this baby bird. Most commonly, the food has been heated in a microwave oven but microwaves do not heat food evenly. Though the temperature of the food is tested and apparently of appropriate temperature, pockets of overly heated food may be present. When the food is syringe or tube fed into the ingluvies, the overheated area remains in contact with and causes thermal burn of the ingluvies. Once the burn has healed and the scab falls off, a fistula remains. In many cases the owner does not notice the original injury and only becomes aware of the problem when food spills from the crop. At this stage, it is not an emergency but is very frightening to most owners.
iii. Surgical management is usually postponed until the patient is stable and the wound has matured. In some cases the demarcation between viable and non-viable tissue is readily apparent. In others it may be difficult to distinguish healthy tissue from revitalized tissue. It generally takes 3–5 days from the time of injury for the demarcation to mature. Once it is obvious, the eschar is removed along with any scar tissue uniting the wall of the ingluvies to the skin. The ingluvies is dissected away from the skin to allow the two structures to be closed as separate tissues. The ingluvies is closed in an inverting pattern, if possible, to allow serosa-to-serosa contact. The skin is closed over the crop as a separate layer. In cases with severe damage and necrosis of the ingluvies, every effort is made to maintain the longitudinal integrity of the oesophagus. Resection and anastomosis of the oesophagus and ingluvies are not recommended as the incidence of stricture is much greater. An oesophageal feeding tube may be placed in cases of extensive tissue loss to serve as a stent around which the oesophagus may heal. This will also allow the patient to receive alimentation during the healing period without stressing the repair.

129 The sample demonstrates septate, branching hyphae indicative of a mycotic infection involving the respiratory tract. The characteristics of the hyphae are compatible with those of *Aspergillus* sp.

130 The radiograph **130** is taken during clinical assessment of a Lanner falcon (*Falco biarmicus*) that has been presented to you as a second opinion case, having been suffering from bumblefoot for several weeks. What are the relevant clinical findings on the radiograph and what therapy would you advise?

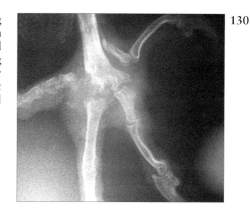

130

131 A 1.3 kg, green-winged macaw (*Ara chloroptera*) was presented with a complaint of feather loss on the distal end of the right wing. A feather cyst had been removed from this area three months earlier. The physical examination revealed a thickened, yellow, friable skin on the dorsal aspect of the right metacarpus. A contact smear was made from an excisional biopsy of the abnormal appearing skin.

i. What is the cytodiagnosis based upon the findings illustrated in **131a, b**?
ii. What is the most likely cause of this condition and how is it treated?

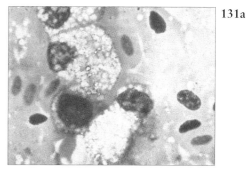

131a

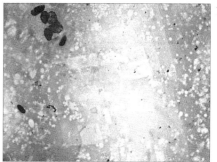

131b

132 i. How does the oviduct appear in a mature, sexually active female bird?
ii. What function do the various sections of the oviduct have in forming the egg?

130 This radiograph shows marked osteomyelitis of the lateral and medial trochlea of the distal tarsometatarsus, as well as the proximal phalanges digits 2 and 3. As such, the bird is classified as suffering from class IV to V bumblefoot, i.e. where there is physical damage to bone or deeper structures of the foot with possible loss of functional use of the foot. The radiograph should be considered concurrently with a clinical assessment. Success rates for treatments of bumblefoot of this severity are very poor. Treatment would comprise extensive surgery, supportive and weight redistributive dressings on both feet and the implantation of antibiotic-impregnated polymethylmethacrylate beads, together with long-term – at least 30 days – parenteral antibiotics. However, the prognosis is grave and euthanasia should be advised prior to further therapy in this case.

131 i. The cytology reveals numerous macrophages, multinucleated giant cell and cholesterol crystals. This is compatible with cutaneous xanthomatosis.
ii. The exact aetiology of xanthomatosis is not known. Cutaneous xanthomatosis can be found anywhere on the body and often overlie neoplasms, such as lipomas, or found in areas of previous trauma and haemorrhage. High fat diets have also been considered to be a predisposing condition for this disorder. Cutaneous xanthomatosis is characterized by numerous lipid-laden macrophages, multinucleated giant cells, and cholesterol crystals. It is likely in this case that this foreign body-like reaction resulted from haemorrhage in the affected area associated with the feather cyst surgery. All the blood components, except cholesterol, were reabsorbed. The cholesterol remaining in the skin acted like a foreign body resulting in the cellular response and the xanthomatosis; there is no specific medical treatment for this condition. Frequently, the affected skin tends to spread and surgical excision is the only course of action available. Correction of a poor diet should also be made.

132 i. Only the left oviduct develops and differentiates in most avian species. The oviduct appears as a convoluted tube lying just ventral to the kidneys and generally above and to the left of the intestines. The oviduct has five identifiable areas: the infundibulum, magnum, isthmus, uterus and vagina. The uterus can weigh as much as 6% of the bird's bodyweight during the breeding season and shrink to less than 1% of body mass during non-breeding periods. During reproductively active periods, as much as 20% of cardiac output will go to the ovary and oviduct.
ii. In most psittacines, the egg will be laid less than 24 hours after ovulation. The infundibulum has two sections, a funnel followed by a tubular portion. As the ovum is expelled from the ovary, it moves to the funnel where fertilization occurs. The tubular portion of the infundibulum is also called the chalaziferous region. (In the brown kiwi, both ovaries but only the left oviduct develop. The funnel portion of the infundibulum becomes very wide and receives ova expelled from either ovary.) The magnum is characterized by enlarged mucosal folds – excretion of cells in this area forms the white of the egg. The next part of the oviduct is the isthmus – glandular cells in the isthmus produce the shell membrane. There is no distinct anatomical boundary between the isthmus and the uterus but there is a distinct functional difference. The tubular cells of the uterus lay down the eggshell. The final portion of the uterus is the S-shaped vagina which contains powerful smooth muscles. Sperm-host glands – the main location of sperm storage in the female reproductive tract – are found in the vagina. In immature waterfowl and some other species, there is a membrane covering the oviduct at the cloaca. This membrane breaks down at sexual maturity.

133 What does **133** show concerning the beak of this 14-day-old cockatoo chick?

- The beak is normal.
- It shows bradygnathism, which must be corrected.
- It will correct itself as the bird matures.
- It is only held abnormally due to the young age of the chick.

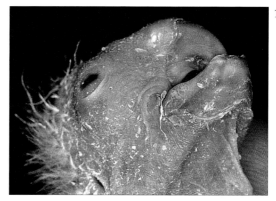

134 This insect (**134**) is known to transmit which disease of avicultural importance?

- Herpesvirus.
- *Sarcocystis falcatula.*
- *E. coli.*
- *Leucocytozoan* sp.

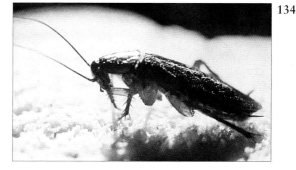

135 A young, hand-reared eclectus parrot is presented with an annular toe deformity (**135**). The distal portion of the toe is warm but oedematous. What treatment is indicated?

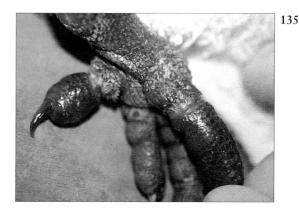

133 This chick shows severe bradygnathism of the maxilla. Due to the severe nature of the defect in this bird, it must be corrected to prevent the beak from growing into the mouth. In mild cases, the bird can move the tip of the maxilla into the mandible and may hold it there at times. To correct this defect in a small chick, the inside of the tip (the caudal surface) of the maxilla can be trimmed with cuticle clippers and the tip pulled cranially with each feeding, or as frequently as needed for correction. Also examine the mandible; if it is compressed laterally so that it is narrow and/or pointed in front, it should be manipulated so that it becomes flatter in front and more spread out at the sides. If the defect is not corrected before the beak becomes hardened it should be corrected by applying an acrylic extension to the tip of the maxilla.

134 *Sarcocystis falcatula.* Sarcocystosis occurs when a parrot ingests the infectious sporocysts of sarcocystosis which are shed in the faeces of the Virginia opossum. Cockroaches have been proven capable of physical transmission by consuming opossum faeces and then transporting the sporocysts to the bird's cage. The cockroach may be eaten by the bird or may contaminate the food with their faeces. The life cycle of *S. falcatula* requires a definitive host (the Virginia opossum) and an intermediate host (the grackle or cowbird). Opossums are infected by eating an infected cowbird or grackle which has *Sarcocystis* encysted in the muscles. Old World psittacine birds – such as cockatoos, and African and Asian parrots – are susceptible to an acute fatal disease characterized by severe pulmonary congestion.

135 Eclectus. African grey parrots and macaws are most often afflicted by this condition. Some annular toe deformities – also called 'constricted toe syndrome' – if mild may be managed medically by increasing the ambient humidity, massaging the toe and providing hot compresses, as well as removing any obvious constricting bands. In cases where the constriction is deep and is causing severe oedema or necrosis, surgery is indicated.

Isoflurane anaesthesia should be used and additional care taken in relation to the risks of hypothermia – as neonates are at greater risk – during the procedure. Apply a tourniquet on the leg to control intraoperative bleeding, and utilising magnification and the constricting band, should be removed. Having freshened up the tissues on either side of the constriction, simple interrupted sutures of a non-absorbable monofilament material are placed. A hydroactive dressing is applied after surgery to prevent scab formation, which could in itself cause a further constriction.

It is recommended that the chick is kept at a higher than normal humidity and not placed on substrate that might desiccate the feet. The ambient humidity should be maintained at at least 50%. Lotion-impregnated facial tissues work well as a container substrate to keep the feet moist and subtle. Sutures should be removed after 7–10 days.

Serious constrictions – or cases where presentation has been delayed – may require digit amputation. Multiple annular toe deformities may occur, necessitating surgery on several toes at the same time. If surgery is performed aseptically, postoperative antibiotics should not be necessary. If the toe is necrotic, amputation alone is indicated.

136 Alleviation of pain is an important aspect of emergency and critical care. Which of the following criteria is helpful in determining if a patient is in pain?

• Would an analogous lesion be painful to a human?
• What degree of tissue trauma has occurred?
• Is the patient exhibiting an adverse response to the lesion?
• All of the above.

137 When opening the air cell of a suspected dead Canada goose egg, you encounter the situation shown in **137**.
i. What is the aetiological agent that produces the pathology seen in this egg?
ii. In addition to the lesion pictured, what are the other signs of this particular causative agent found in embryos or newly hatched birds?
iii. What is required for positive diagnosis?
iv. What are recommended treatments and preventive measures for this problem?

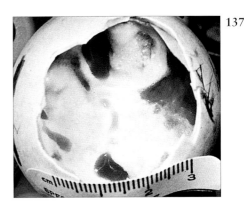

137

138 Lumbosacral plexus. The paired kidneys of birds are divided into three divisions: cranial, middle and caudal (**138a**). What major structure will be revealed if the kidneys of the yellow-crowned Amazon parrot (*Amazona ochrecephala*) are dissected away? How can disease in this area cause paralysis of the legs?

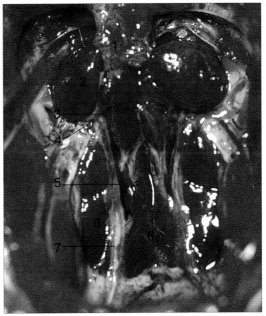

138a

1 Adrenal gland
2 Cranial division of the kidney
3 Common iliac vein
4 External iliac vein
5 Caudal renal vein
6 Caudal division of the kidney
7 Urates in the ureter

136 The correct choice is the last one. Symptoms and signs may indicate pain including change in temperament (aggressive or passive), appearance of being uncomfortable (unable to rest), decrease in normal activity, especially grooming (often exhibited as fluffing or a reluctance to perch), anorexia, lameness, or dropped wing, guarding the back or splinting of the abdomen, and biting or chewing at the surgical site, sutures or bandage. Rolling or thrashing may be a sign of severe pain but must be differentiated from seizures or rough recovery from anaesthesia, especially if ketamine has been used. Procedures likely to be painful include burns, crushing, trauma (especially those injuries involving long bones and large muscle masses), beak trauma, and abrasions or bruising of distal extremities, especially the scaled skin of the feet.

137 i. The figure shows a fungal infection growing in the air cell of the membrane. The most common aetiological agents producing such growth are *Aspergillus* sp., typically *A. fumigatus* but occasionally *A. flavus*.
ii. Embryos may die before hatching or be weak and dyspnoeic after hatching. Occasionally, nervous system problems or diarrhoea are found in birds that survive to hatch. Post-mortem findings include bronchial or tracheal plugs, air cell plaques or small yellow nodules in the lungs.
iii. Cultures of lesions on the air cell membrane, lungs, air sacs or air passages are collected for positive identification.
iv. There is currently no recommended treatment for eggs infected with aspergillosis; efforts should be concentrated on prevention. Aspergillosis can be a serious problem in forced-air incubators. Always clean and fumigate incubators and hatchers between batches of eggs and operate an 'all in, all out' policy. Eggs should be examined – weighed; candled; examined for cracks – at regular intervals. Dead eggs should be removed at once as contamination of viable eggs by dead *Aspergillus*-infected eggs can occur. Eggs from damp or wet nests should not be incubated. UV sterilization of eggs may be used prior to incubation, as may sanitizing dips or washes.

138b

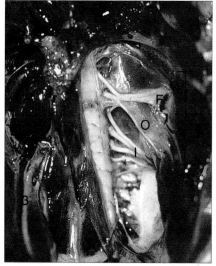

138 The kidneys lie in the renal fossa formed by the pelvis, which is fused to the synsacrum. Between the fossa and the kidney is the lumbosacral plexus forming the femoral nerve (F), obturator nerve (O) and the ilioischiadic nerve (I) (**138b**). Because of the close proximity of the nerves to the kidneys, nephritis can frequently cause neuritis; likewise, renal neoplasia will cause pressure on the nerves. In both cases the legs can become paralysed.

1 Cranial division
2 Intermediate divison
3 Caudal division
4 Lumbosacral plexus

139 This five-year-old male budgerigar is presented with lameness and articular swelling of the foot and intertarsal joint (**139**). Through the skin, whitish material can be seen. What is your differential diagnosis and how can you confirm this? What is your therapeutic approach?

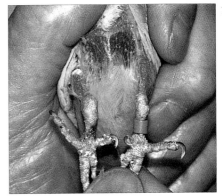

140 A client presents a somnolent, emaciated cockatiel exhibiting diarrhoea. Diagnostic work-up included faecal examination. Large numbers of this ovum (**140**) were visualized.
i. Name the species or type of ovum.
ii. How would you treat this infection?
iii. How would you prevent this infection?

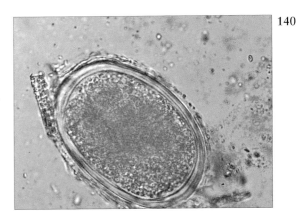

141 Radiosurgical incision (**141**). What are five principal factors that control the amount of lateral heat damage occurring in a radiosurgical incision?

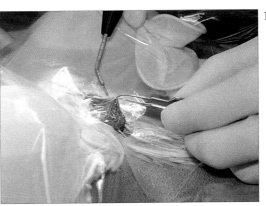

139 The differential diagnosis would be articular gout or bacterial arthritis. To confirm a diagnosis, material can be collected for further examination. In articular gout the material looks macroscopically like toothpaste. The presence of urate can be confirmed by performing the murexide test: a drop of nitric acid is mixed with a small amount of the suspected material on a slide and dried by evaporation in a Bunsen flame. After cooling, one drop of concentrated ammonia is added. In the presence of urate, a mauve colour will develop. Alternatively a polarizing microscope can be used to identify urate crystals.

In bacterial arthritis, bacteria and white blood cells can be identified in a smear for cytological examination. By culture, the bacteria can be isolated and identified.

In articular gout, a chronic renal disorder or a high protein diet should be suspected. Fluid balance and the vitamin A status should be checked (history and physical examination) and corrected when necessary. A low protein diet is recommended. Treatment with allopurinol and probenecid is controversial and has been used successfully by some clinicians. High doses of allopurinol have been shown to be able to induce gout in red-tailed hawks. Probenecid is contraindicated in birds. In man the uricosuric action of probenicid is based on reduced absorption of uric acid in the tubuli although glomerular secretion is also slightly inhibited. Since birds lack the reabsorptive mechanism for uric acid, and uric acid excretion is mainly based on active secretion by the tubuli, the net effect of the use of probenicid in birds might even be a reduced uric acid excretion. Bacterial pododermatitis should be treated with a combination of antibiotics and surgery after antimicrobial sensitivity testing.

140 i. *Ascaridia* sp.; roundworm ovum.
ii. Pyrantel pamoate 4.5 mg kg^{-1} repeat 10 days; ivermectin 200 mg kg^{-1} i.m.; fenbendazole 25 mg kg^{-1} p.o.
iii. In flock or flight situations, separate the birds from the ground by using suspended flights. Monitor faeces regularly.

141 The five principal factors are:

- Frequency – it has been shown that 3.8–4.0 MHz is the optimum frequency for tissue incision. This frequency, with its short waveform, provides a precision focus of the energy in a minimal area.
- Power setting – if the power setting is too high, there is excessive sparking and lateral heat damage. If it is too low, the 'electrode' drags and actually tears tissue, causing excessive lateral heat and damage.
- Waveform – if the waveform is fully filtered, it is less pulsatile in nature and there is minimal lateral heat.
- Electrode size – the greater the non-insulated surface area of the electrode, the more energy is radiated from it and therefore more lateral heat is generated. A very small diameter fine-wire electrode provides an incision with the least lateral heat damage to adjacent tissue.
- Time – the longer the tissue is exposed to the energy, the more lateral heat is created in the tissue. A smooth rapid stroke is necessary to minimise tissue damage. The operator should not return to cut the same tissue within 7 seconds if using a fine, straight wire electrode or within 15 seconds if using a loop electrode.

142 During the spring breeding season, a breeder reports that on their lake, during the previous week, they had observed some sick migratory waterfowl. The birds showed signs of ataxia, bloody nasal discharge and acute death. Now, one of the breeder's Muscovy ducks is showing signs of neck weakness, drooped wings, bloody diarrhoea and some have died (142a).

i. What are the differential diagnoses based on the clinical history as presented?
ii. What diagnostic tests should be performed?
iii. What treatment or preventive measures can be suggested?

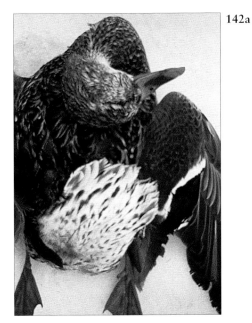
142a

143 A flock of budgerigars are examined; they have a history of unthriftiness, diarrhoea and weight loss. The stools are light green and pea soup consistency. A direct smear of fresh faeces yields these organisms (143).

i. Identify the organism.
ii. Describe the type of drug used for therapy.
iii. What environmental measures would you recommend?

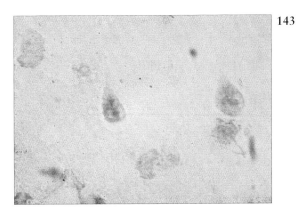
143

144 What criteria may be monitored during gaseous surgical anaesthesia?

142b 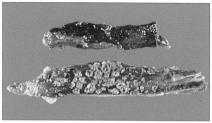 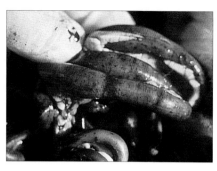 142c

142 i. Differentials include DVE, DVH, pasturellosis, necrotic enteritis and toxicosis, e.g. lead.

ii. Initial diagnostics tests should include necropsy and histopathology. At necropsy, petechiae and ecchymotic lesions were observed in the myocardium and visceral organs. Elevated white/yellow plaques were observed under the tongue, oesophagus and intestinal lining (**142b**). Haemorrhagic annular bands were observed in the small intestine (**142c**). These lesions are consistent with DVE and may be confirmed on histopathology and viral isolation.

iii. Management includes removal of affected birds and vaccination of captive populations where possible. Transmission is direct or indirect with an incubation period of 3–7 days. Muscovy ducks are very sensitive to this virus and call ducks are resistant. As the infection is caused by a herpesvirus, any surviving birds may become persistently infected and virus-shedding birds. The collection should be vaccinated the following year two weeks prior to the disease outbreak as experienced this year.

143 i. *Giardia* sp.

ii. Substitute imidazoles – metronidazole; carnidazole; ronidazole; ipronanidazole – are most frequently used to treat avian giardiasis. Recurrence is common, due to either incomplete cure or reinfection.

iii. This organism is susceptible to desiccation. Well-drained aviaries are less likely to provide a substrate for the transmission of *Giardia* sp.

144 Reflexes that can be evaluated are: (1) muscle tone (jaw tone); (2) palpebral and corneal reflexes; (3) painful stimuli (toe pinch); (4) respiratory depth and rate, or cardiac rate; (5) Doppler, pulse oximetry and capnography are useful supportive techniques but do not give such an accurate assessment of the bird's physiological status. The first, second and third reflexes are difficult to access, difficult to evaluate and unreliable, although of these the corneal reflex is the most useful. The most accurate visual method of determining the plane of anaesthesia is to observe the thoracic excursions (movements). The respiratory rate and depth must be observed. For correct surgical anaesthesia, the respirations should be deep, slow and regular. If the bird is too light the rate will be rapid and irregular, if too deep the respirations will be shallow (see table below on monitoring planes of anaesthesia).

	Light	*Surgical*	*Deep*
Respirations:	Deep	Deep	Shallow
	Rapid	slow	Slow
	Irregular	Regular	Regular

145 A freshly imported mynah bird was introduced with a history of respiratory distress, vomiting and weight loss. Besides physical examination, laparoscopy was performed. The tip of the endoscope is within the abdominal air sac (145).

i. Identify organ (1).

ii. What has to be kept in mind before performing a laparoscopy in mynah birds?

iii. What further diagnostic procedures would you perform?

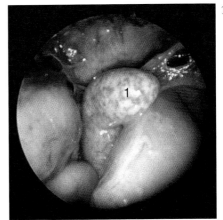

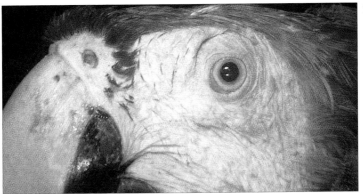

146 Which is correct? This green-winged macaw (146):

• Is normal.
• Looks old and has lost the elasticity to the skin.
• Has a severe sinusitis that has resulted in collapsed sinuses.
• Is dehydrated.

147 Why should different age groups be segregated within a pigeon loft?

145 i. The organ is the spleen, which is bean shaped and more elongated in finches and pigeons. The colour should be purple to brownish-red – as in psittacines – and it should be half the size in a mynah bird.

ii. Remember: 'Will the patient's suspected problem cause procedural difficulties during examination?' Ascites, for example, which is often seen in mynah birds due to iron storage disease (haemochromatosis), increases the potential risk of the procedure tremendously.

iii. A diagnosis cannot be made by visualization of the organs alone. The discoloration and enlargement of the spleen is often seen in connection with septicaemia.

During the endoscopic examination special attention should be given to the liver, air sacs and kidneys. If the liver is enlarged, a biopsy of it would be a good choice to diagnose haemochromatosis.

If air sacculitis can be seen, a Gram stain and/or culture of a swab taken directly under endoscopic control would give further information. In this case, air sacculitis and splenomegaly are seen. A swab was taken from the air sac for culture and enrofloxacin was administered i.m. following the procedure. *Pseudomonas* sp. was isolated from the air sac and faecal swab. The bird recovered in three days.

The symptomatic diagnosis was air sacculitis and splenomegaly. The aetiological diagnosis was *Pseudomonas* sp. infection.

146 The macaw has severe bacterial sinusitis, causing a collapse of the sinuses. This condition typically responds well to antibiotic therapy based on culture and sensitivity testing. It is associated with copious amounts of mucous exudate in the sinuses and requires vigorous flushing with large quantities of saline through the sinuses to dislodge the exudate. This bird was flushed with 60 ml of saline through each nostril daily until the sinuses returned to normal. The exudate was flushed out of the choana harmlessly. The condition is most often seen in recently imported macaws. This problem occurs especially with *Pseudomonas* or *Bordetella* sp. infections.

147 The principle of segregated age groups is well known in poultry. Husbandry and environmental requirements vary with respect to age, as do levels of maternal and acquired immunity. Mixing birds of differing ages can lead to the exposure of some birds to pathogens to which they have no immunity. Some fanciers manipulate the breeding flock so that young are produced over a prolonged period. If young of different ages cannot be segregated, an extended breeding season should not be used.

148 i. An orphan wild bird is found and brought to your clinic by a member of the public. What advice would you give to the person who has presented the chick?
ii. What particular problems are associated with rearing young wild birds?
iii. What are the advantages and disadvantages of rearing such orphans in groups?
iv. What is imprinting? If you have to rear a chick by itself, what actions can you take to reduce the likelihood of imprinting?
v. Can imprinted birds be released into the wild? Why?

149 A Moluccan cockatoo (*Cacatua moluccensis*) – residing in a hotel display – was found dead. The veterinarian performed a post-mortem examination. Samples included organ impression smears to be stained with Gimenez for chlamydial inclusion bodies. The slide was examined under high power (**149**).
i. What do you see?
ii. Where did this creature come from?
iii. Does this finding explain the cause of death?
iv. How would you treat this on an ante-mortem basis?

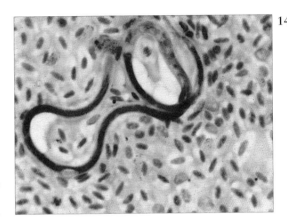

149

150 During laparoscopy of a seagull (**150**), this white structure could be identified on the intestine (arrowed). What is your diagnosis?

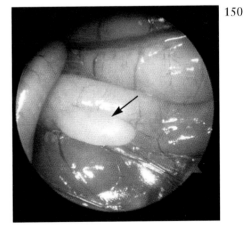

150

148 i. Whenever a so-called orphaned wild bird is brought to the clinic, the intended Good Samaritan should be encouraged to take it back to the site where it was found (in some countries or states this is illegal). Birds have a very poor sense of smell so the handling of the chick by humans will not upset the mother who is still likely to be in the area and will return to her calling chick to feed it. The chick should be placed in an elevated position with some protection from predators and the elements.

ii. Neonates are susceptible to the effects of starvation and chilling (especially altricial chicks), particularly since the gut is described as being immune incompetent, having a very poorly developed bacterial flora until after 14 days. Young of most species are likely to become imprinted on humans (the provider of food), the food and the nest construction in which they are raised. The imprinting on to humans and on to an unnatural diet are deleterious if the bird is destined for release into the wild. Imprinting on to a novel nest site has been used to an advantage in the protection of a wild bird population, where the bird's natural nest site or situation has become short in supply, e.g. pine trees of a certain height. Birds may be trained to recognize a new nesting site, e.g. telegraph poles, thereby increasing the species' future breeding opportunities.

iii. The advantage of rearing orphans in groups of their own is that imprinting on to humans can be avoided. The disadvantage is that numerous young, potentially infected chicks are all mixed together, hence generating a significant disease risk. However, it is believed that group rearing is, on balance, to be recommended.

iv. Imprinting is the recognition of the food provider as parent, and likewise food and nest site as being natural. If a neonate *has* to be reared on its own, then the bird should not see the human face or hand but instead be puppet-fed by a gloved hand through the side of a box.

v. Imprinted birds cannot be released into the wild as, when they reach sexual maturity, they may seek a human as a mate. Also, they may attack members of their own species who make advances to them and they may occupy a breeding site or nest which, if they are in short supply, might prevent another potentially productive pair from breeding.

149 i. The preparation appears negative for chlamydial inclusions; a microfilaria is visible.

ii. Blood-sucking insects are the source of the infection. Mostly non-pathogenic adults reside in subcutaneous and serosal areas.

iii. Filarids rarely cause clinical disease but occasional aberrant lesions can cause death.

iv. There is no effective therapy available that will clear microfilaria and adults.

150 Although many psittacine species have no caecum, in most other bird species the large intestine consists of a paired caecum and a short, straight rectum. The anatomy of the caecum varies among species. The white structure is a caecum.

151 What is the most likely cause of the lesions on the face of this blue and gold macaw (151)?

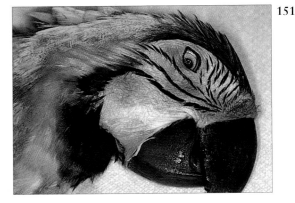

- Trauma from fighting.
- Age spots.
- Poxvirus lesions.
- Bee stings.

152 The vocal virtuosity of birds stems from the structure of their unusual and powerful vocal apparatus, the syrinx (152).
i. Can you describe the functional anatomical base of the sound production?
ii. Which birds have well developed syringeal muscles and what is their specific role?
iii. What is the effect of a needle puncture of the interclavicular air sac in respect to sound production? Explain.

First bronchial half-ring
Semilunar membrane
Second bronchial half-ring
Internal labium — Pessulus
External labium — External tympaniform membrane
Third bronchial half-ring
Internal tympaniform membrane
Interclavicular air sac

iv. Describe two methods of devoicing highly vocal male birds. Comment on the efficacy and safety of each.

153 During the summer a number of waterfowl have been found dead on the shore or 'paralysed' (153) at a city park. The lake is shallow and heavily overgrown with foliage.
i. What is your preliminary diagnosis and how would you confirm it?
ii. What conditions lead to this problem?
iii. What is the best treatment, control and prevention plan?

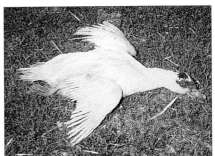

151–153: Answers

151 This unfortunate macaw was attacked by a swarm of bees which stung the bird at least 25 times. Despite rapid therapy with dexamethasone and antihistamines, the bird developed a rapidly fatal anaphylaxis. The lesions appeared shortly after the incident and the bird died within 2 hours.

152 i. Contraction of the thoracic and abdominal muscles forces air from the main air sacs through the bronchi to the syrinx. On each side of the syrinx is a thin, glass-clear membrane, the *m. tympaniformis interna*. Sound is caused by the vibration of the air column as air passes through the narrow (syringeal) passageways, which are bounded on opposite sides by corresponding projections called the internal labium and external labium. Vibration of the internal tympaniform membrane, regulated by its mass, internal tension, and protrusion into the adjacent air column, determine the sound characteristics. Pressure in the interclavicular air sac pushes the thin membrane into the bronchial air space, into position for vibration and creation of sounds. Many birds can stimulate the two sides of the syrinx independently and thus can sing two songs simultaneously.
ii. Syringeal muscles control syringeal function by changing the tension of the tympaniform membrane as a bird sings. These muscles are especially well developed in passerines and psittacines.
iii. A needle puncture of the interclavicular air sac prevents build-up of the pressure needed to move the tympaniform membranes, thereby rendering a bird voiceless. Devoicing has often been attempted by causing thermal or caustic damage to the internal tympaniform membrane. This procedure carries a high degree of risk, and the devoicing may not be effective in the long term. An alternative method is the surgical castration of the male bird; castration is simpler, less life-threatening and the effects can be permanent if the ablation of the testicle is complete.

153 i. Avian botulism – limber neck; alkali duck disease – is diagnosed based on identification of *Clostridium botulinum* type C toxin, which does not affect mammals. This toxin is most commonly found in maggots on carcasses. Serum toxin analysis or mouse inoculation neutralization tests confirm the diagnosis. Birds suffer an acute flaccid paralysis of the voluntary muscles, often occurring in mid swim, leading to death by drowning.
ii. Outbreaks occur in hot weather, due to alkali and anaerobic conditions arising, often in stagnant water. As the water temperature rises, oxygen levels fall, the latter possibly being exacerbated by decaying organic matter in the water. Fish and invertebrate carcasses act as a substrate for clostridial spores and hence toxin production, the toxin may then become concentrated in maggots that are feeding on the carcass.
iii. If the bird can still walk but not fly, good nursing and supportive care will often be effective. If the bird can swim but not walk, the prognosis is not so good, but it may recover. Therapy involves oral fluids with activated charcoal and bismuth. Antitoxins are not proven to be effective and they are expensive. Control involves the removal of all carcasses from the water, as well as the removal of decaying vegetable material. The toxin is stable in water and the area of water will typically remain contaminated until the increased water flow caused by autumn storms, for example, washes the toxin away. Water flow and oxygenation should be improved if possible. Vaccination yearly with type C toxoid is helpful.

154 i. The bird in 154, from a collection of six, is presented with ocular and nasal discharge and watery green diarrhoea. What is the first and most important differential diagnosis? How would you confirm your suspicions?
ii. Some tests give false negatives. Why?
iii. If the diagnosis is positive, state the pros and cons of therapy as you would discuss them with the owner.
iv. What further action should be taken apart from treatment of the bird?
v. What therapeutic options are available for this bird?
vi. How would you confirm that the infection has been cleared from the bird's system?

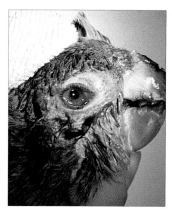
154

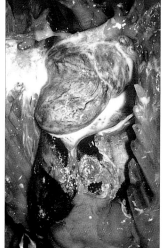
155

155 This lesion (155) was found at necropsy of a cocka-too.
i. What are the primary dif-ferential diagnoses?
ii. What is the distinguishing histological feature of the con-dition?
iii. What is the pathogenesis of the lesion?

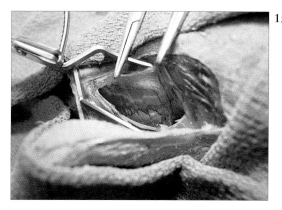
156

156 Spaying a bird (156).
i. Describe the approach.
ii. What is the correct name for the procedure?
iii. What is done with the ovary?
iv. Which blood vessel should be clamped?
v. What is done with the ventral ligament of the uterus and oviduct and why?
vi. Where is the uterus ligated prior to its removal and what happens if too much uterus is left with the patient?
vii. How does this procedure affect the bird's reproductive behaviour?

154 i. For psittacosis confirm diagnosis by PCR on blood or faeces and ELISA on faeces or serology. Paired samples are often required for serology.
ii. Blood and faecal PCR and faecal ELISA can give false negatives as the organism is often latent, during which stages shedding may not occur, hence the tests are then negative.
iii. If therapy is to be carried out, the risk of zoonosis during initial treatment and the risk to other birds in the collection should be considered. The treatment must be continued for 40–45 days with doxycycline or 21–45 days with enrofloxacin. The clinician and owner must consider the likelihood of complete eradication of the organism – especially in a collection of birds – as well as the potential for recurrence and the inability to prove eradication of the organism.
iv. The owner must be warned of the zoonotic potential; the health of his family and staff should be verified. Other birds in the collection should be screened and treated if positive, or treated anyway if, for example, they share the same air space.
v. Enrofloxacin for 21–45 days or doxycyline for 40–45 days. The latter may be given as long-acting injections (Vibravenous) every 5–7 days although there is a risk of associated myositis, or twice daily medication in food if the birds will take a soft mix, or impregnated pellets.
vi. Following treatment, faecal samples should be bulked, i.e. a sample from each bird daily for a 3-day period and tested. There is no way of ever proving a bird is cleared of latent infection. However, the clinician may advise periodic serological testing, a gradually falling titre being indicative of effective therapy and the absence of recrudescence.

155 i. This is a case of severe visceral urate deposition – gout. Differential diagnoses: infectious pericarditis and epicarditis, as well as severe myocardial mineralization.
ii. Histologically there is deposition of amorphous urates in the pericardial sac, the epicardium and within the fluid found in the pericardial sac.
iii. Severe visceral gout is usually secondary to severe renal disease but it may also occur due to metabolic disorders of protein metabolism or severe dehydration.

156 i. A left lateral coeliotomy approach is being used for this procedure. The skin incision extends from the pubic bone to the level of the third from last rib. The last two ribs are transected just dorsal to the junction between the sternal and vertebral ribs following coagulation of the intercostal blood vessels. A retractor is positioned between the cut ends of the ribs to enable visualization of coelomic structures. The abdominal air sac will need to be entered to access the female reproductive tract. The intestines and ventriculus are retracted medially and ventrally to allow visualization of the kidney dorsomedially. The ovary is located at the cranial division of the kidney.
ii. Salpingohysterectomy as the oviduct (salpinx) and uterus are removed, but not the ovary.
iii. It is not feasible to remove the ovary in birds.
iv. The cranial oviductal artery and vein are clamped prior to transection.
v. It is broken down by blunt or sharp dissection. There are no significant blood vessels in it and it must be broken down to allow visualization of the dorsal ligament that contains the blood vessels supplying the oviduct and uterus.
vi. The uterus is ligated or clipped with a haemostatic clip at the vagina or as close to the cloaca as possible. If too much uterine tissue is left, the feedback loop may not be disrupted and the bird might ovulate yolks into the coelomic cavity.
vii. Birds retain their reproductive behaviour but do not lay eggs.

157 Which of the following is correct? 'Shock' as defined on a physiologic basis:

- Occurs in birds just as it does in mammals.
- Does not occur in birds as it does in mammals.
- Occurs in birds as a result of hypovolaemia but not as a result of hypotension.
- Occurs in birds as a result of hypotension but not as a result of hypovolaemia.

158 The opacity in the eye of this macaw (158) is due to which of the following?

- A cataract associated with ageing.
- A corneal scar secondary to previous poxvirus infection.
- This is a normal eye.
- Corneal oedema secondary to uveitis.

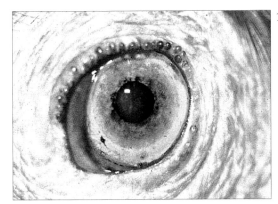

158

159 A canary breeder keeps about 30 birds in one large, unscreened aviary. Since the onset of spring the breeder has experienced four deaths in adult birds. She presents a clinically ill canary for diagnosis and treatment. You take a blood sample and find the following (159).
i. What are the objects in the erythrocytes?
ii. How would you treat this problem?
iii. How would you prevent the problem?

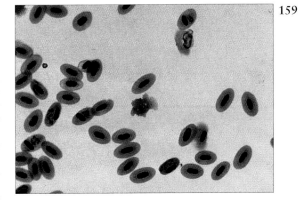

159

157–159: Answers

157 The second choice is correct. Shock, as defined in mammals, does not occur in birds. That is to say that birds do not develop lactic-acidosis caused by cellular hypoxia that progresses to peripheral circulatory failure and the pooling of blood in terminal circulatory beds in small vessels. General failure of the circulation does occur, however, because of hypovolaemia and heart failure and is thought to occur because of sepsis. It is the pathogenesis at the tissue and cellular levels that differs.

Birds react to hypovolaemia and hypotension in much the same manner as other animals. Reduced blood pressure causes an increase in precapillary resistance. This is associated with an increase in catecholamines, primarily norepinephrine. This change, in chickens, is not associated with a carotid sinus baroreceptor as it is in mammals. Birds tolerate blood loss better than most animals. In a study of animals bled at a rate of 1% body weight per hour, mammals and non-flying avian species were out-performed by flying birds. Some pigeons survived removal of blood equalling 9% of their body weight – equal to their total blood volume – before significant mortality occurred. This illustrates the degree that birds can move fluids from their interstitial space into their circulation. The fluid movement results in haemodilution. Decreases in haematocrit, haemoglobin and plasma proteins affect osmolarity and osmotic pressure.

FFAs, which are the major source of energy for avian tissues, are similarly stimulated by the release of catecholamines. There is little breakdown of adipose tissue for this purpose. During fasting, nearly 90% of the mobilized lipids are stored in the liver. Paradoxically, the liver converts FFAs into ketoacids rather than triglycerides. Whether this is due to a fatty acid overload or as a preferred metabolic pathway is yet to be determined. Prostaglandins, which play an important role in haemorrhage in mammals, have not been shown to be involved in the bird's (i.e. chicken's) reaction to hypovolaemia or hypotension.

Hypovolaemia and hypotension may result in acidosis in birds. Poor oxygenation can be assumed to occur but lactic-acidosis due to the anaerobic formation of lactate from pyruvate does not occur, glycogen stores are not depleted nor does lipolysis take place. In critically ill patients, acidosis may result as a consequence of FFAs used for energy rather than incomplete lipid oxygenation or anaerobic formation of lactate due to the poor oxygenation of tissues.

158 The opacity is in the lens and is associated with ageing in macaws. Cataracts are common in aged macaws and often occur at 35–45 years old. The cataract may be surgically removed, preferably by phacoemulsification. Careful surgery will return sight to a blind eye so long as retinal function is normal. The eye will be aphacic – have no lens – hence close focusing is not normal due to the lost accommodative function of the lens. After a few weeks' adjustment, sight returns close to functional normality. Hypermature cataracts may degenerate, resulting in phacolytic uveitis with secondary glaucoma and permanent loss of sight.

159 i. The objects are *Plasmodium* sp.
ii. Canary malaria will respond – characterized by a reduced mortality – to the application of chloroquine phosphate at 250 mg per 120 ml water for 14 days.
iii. Prevent exposure to mosquitoes, the main vector for *Plasmodium* sp.

160 A client presents a sulphur-breasted toucan (*Ramphastos sulfuratus*) (160) to you prior to purchasing the bird as a pet. The client is concerned about iron storage disease and wants to be sure the bird is not affected.

i. What is the preferred diagnostic test to correctly assess iron storage disease in this individual?

ii. What other diagnostic tests are available for an accurate assessment of this condition?

iii. How would the preferred diagnostic test be performed?

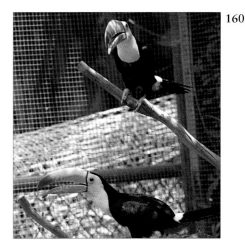

161 What is shown in 161?

- Using physical therapy to correct a lateral deviation of the maxilla – scissor beak deformity – in a macaw chick.
- A restraint technique for macaw chicks.
- A technique to correct a mandibular prognathism.
- Manipulation of the beak for gavage feeding.

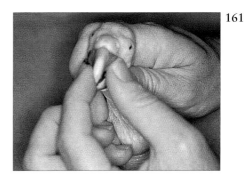

162 The crusty material found on this macaw egg (162) indicates which of the following:

- The egg is fertile.
- The egg was retained excessively long in the oviduct and the hen has an oviduct infection.
- The egg became soiled in the nest.
- This egg is normal for macaws.

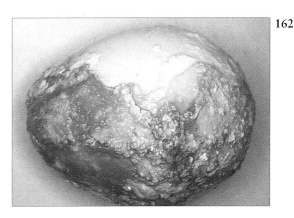

160 i. At the present time the only available test for the accurate ante-mortem diagnosis of haemochromatosis in avian species involves the use of hepatic biopsy. The clinician should contact the pathology laboratory to check the minimum biopsy sample size required. Once a hepatic sample is obtained, submission to a lab for a quantitative analysis for iron concentration – or the histopathological demonstration of changes directly related to iron deposition and the demonstration of iron pigments through the use of special stains – is required.

ii. Currently there are no other accurate diagnostic tests for the ante-mortem diagnosis of haemochromatosis. Previously it was considered that the analysis of iron serum levels and the total iron-binding capacity was a plausible test for the assessment of a bird's hepatic iron level. Subsequent research has unfortunately revealed that this potentially atraumatic methodology is inaccurate in the assessment of a toucan's hepatic iron load. Hence it is necessary to obtain a liver biopsy.

iii. A liver biopsy may be achieved by either of the following methods. Both methods require the use of an anaesthetic, preferably isoflurane. Apart from the usual reasons for increased safety in any avian species, halothane is particularly contraindicated in any case that may have liver pathology. Isoflurane is initially administered by a specially adapted long plastic mask, necessitated by the typically long beak of most ramphastides.

- The first method involves a small abdominal incision, to allow visualization and sampling of the liver. One technique involves an incision site in the right abdominal quadrant, just caudal to the ventral border of the sternum. Through a 10 mm incision, the right lobe of the liver is visualized and a wedge-shaped sample is removed. Excessive bleeding is controlled by the use of an absorbable gel foam. The skin incision is closed. The whole procedure should not exceed 15 minutes.
- The second method involves the use of an endoscope and biopsy forceps to collect a sample. The first method is safer in view of the increased ability to control haemorrhage, should it occur.

161 Scissor beak deformity or lateral deviation of the maxilla is a common developmental abnormality in handfed macaws. It may be associated with feeding techniques but is more commonly associated with irregularity of the mandibular occlusal surface opposing the maxilla. Once the deformity begins, uneven wear of the mandibular occlusal surface aggravates the problem. If observed in small chicks before the beak is calcified, most can be corrected by physical therapy, as in **161**. If the beak is too hard to correct in this way, an acrylic ramp can be placed on the mandible to force the maxilla back into the normal position. In very small chicks, the mandibular occlusal surface should be examined frequently in order to detect irregularities. This malformation is also more common in chicks that are underfed or that have other developmental problems, especially those in which the mandible is laterally compressed and more narrow and pointed at the tip than is normal.

162 The crusty material on this egg was present when the egg was laid. Birds with oviduct infections may retain an egg for an extended period of time and have a build-up of extra calcium, or in this case yolk material, on the surface of the egg.

163 When anaesthetizing and performing surgery on this patient (163), what anatomical and physiological considerations must be understood?

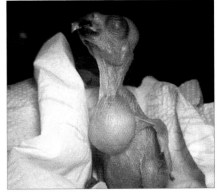

163

164a

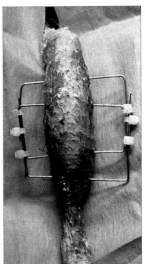

164b

164 The tibiotarsus of a Harris hawk (*Parabuteo unicinctus*), having been repaired using two different methods, is shown in 164a, b.
i. Is this injury common in such birds, when does it occur and what is the cause?
ii. How can this injury be best prevented?
iii. List the pros and cons of each method of fracture repair.

165 You discover this creature (165) crawling on your shirt after working with a group of ostriches.
i. What is this insect?
ii. How can you identify affected birds?
iii. What is the treatment of choice?

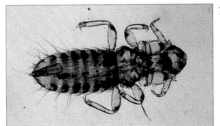

165

163 Anatomical – the glottis and trachea of a neonate or paediatric patient are soft and friable and since the tracheal rings are complete (no ligament), care must be taken when inserting, and particularly when removing, the endotracheal tube. Extreme caution must be taken not to overinflate the cuff. Because oesophageal reflux can be a hazard, the crop should be aspirated and emptied. The fasting of baby birds can cause hypoglycaemia, therefore a fast in excess of 2 hours is potentially lethal and must be avoided.

Physiological – the rate of oxygen consumption is 2–3 times as great as in adult birds. Therefore the oxygen flow rate must be 2–3 times greater, pro rata, for the size of bird, to meet the oxygen demand and avoid excessive CO_2 build-up and hypoxia.

Careful monitoring is essential because bradycardia can be a major problem if undetected. Young patients are less able to compensate for haemorrhage which can result in tachycardia and hypotension. Induction and recovery is more rapid in the neonate than in the adult. Featherless neonates have more difficulty in maintaining core body temperature.

164 i. This is the most common fracture of captive birds of prey. It invariably occurs in the first two weeks that a bird is 'jessed' and tethered to a perch. It arises when the bird 'bates' (flies) away from the perch. When the bird reaches the extremity of the 'jessie', which attaches the bird to the perch, it is suddenly prevented from going further, resulting in a sudden and severe backward force being placed on the legs. The fracture occurs at the junction of the first and second third of the tibiotarsus.
ii. Incidence is reduced if the bird is left in a quiet place where it will not bate. The height of the perch should keep the bird's tail just clear of the ground. The smaller the perch, the shorter the length of the leash which is required. The longer the leash, the greater the speed prior to being stopped and so a greater fracture incidence.
iii. 164a shows a fracture repaired using a single intramedullary pin. The technique gives longitudinal stability but does not prevent longitudinal rotation. The latter can be minimized by stack pinning rather than single pinning, and by the placement of an aluminium finger splint around the tibiotarsus for the first 10 days postoperatively to prevent rotational movement. The proximal end of the pin is situated on the anterior aspect of the stifle joint; if care is not taken with placement or it is not removed after surgery it can cause joint damage. The technique is simple and quick, and rarely gives rise to complications. No foreign material is left *in situ* after healing.

164b shows a full pin fixation technique with two pins below the fracture site and two above. Generally a polyethylene intramedullary drift is used to bridge the fracture site and ensure correct horizontal alignment. The technique takes longer than that shown above and the polyethylene drift is left *in situ* after healing. The placement of the pins as shown in **164b**, through both the medial and lateral soft tissues, can occasionally lead to temporary soft tissue (including nerve) reactions. The great benefit of the technique is that it allows full and normal function of both the stifle and tarsal joints immediately following surgery.

165 i. This is the ostrich louse, *Struthiolipeurus struthionis*.
ii. *S. struthionis* is a chewing louse that feeds on sloughed epidermis and feathers by removing the barbules, thereby making the feathers appear thin and tattered. A diagnosis can be made by observing the eggs (nits) on the barbs along the shaft of the feathers, especially under the wing or crawling on the feathers of the adults.
iii. Treatment consists of monthly applications of 5% carbaryl or 2–4% malathion in either powder or liquid form.

166

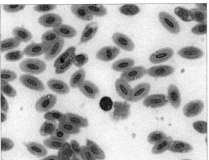

167

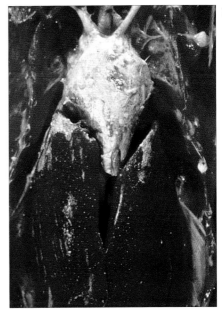

166 i. A blood smear from a saker falcon (*Falco cherrug*) shows erythrocytic intracytoplasmic, small and large, irregular, clear vacuoles surrounded by a slender inner basophilic ring and a slightly wider clear outer ring (**166**). What can these be? You have a choice from:

- Artefacts produced by poor fixation due to methanol contaminated by immersion oil?
- Artefacts due to inadequately stained blood smear, i.e. long-term storage under humid conditions prior to fixation?
- *Babesia shortii* infection?
- *Plasmodium* sp. schizonts?
- *Haemoproteus* sp. gametocytes?

ii. What age group of raptors is most commonly clinically affected by blood parasites?
iii. What clinical signs may be associated with clinical disease caused by blood parasites?
iv. How would you treat clinical disease caused by blood parasites in birds of prey?

167 This bird (**167**) died within a few days of the owner noticing weight loss, poor appetite and polyuria.
i. What is the condition called?
ii. What major nutrient deficiency in seeds could cause this condition in birds?
iii. What nutrients are commonly *thought* to cause this condition but do not?
iv. What are the main known causes of this condition and how is the cause best diagnosed?

168 You are consulted for a second opinion concerning a parrot which was presented with weakness. According to the owner, the first veterinarian diagnosed hypoadrenocorticism – Addison's disease – based on the finding of a plasma potassium concentration of 6.5 mmol l^{-1} (normally 2.1–3.3 mmol l^{-1}) and no response to the ACTH stimulation test. The first veterinarian prescribed life-long therapy with mineralocorticoids. How would you react to this request for a second opinion?

166 i. They are caused by *Babesia shortii* infection.
ii. Immature birds of prey are at a greater risk of heavy infection by blood parasites, leading on occasions to clinical disease.
iii. Most haematozoa infections in birds of prey are mild (affecting less than 2% of erythrocytes) and therefore asymptomatic. However, clinical signs in heavily infected birds (greater than 5–8%) include weight loss, dyspnoea, vomiting, bright green mutes, lethargy, icterus and anorexia. Heavy infections with haematozoa, but in particular *Haemoproteus* sp., *Plasmodium* sp. and *Babesia* sp. can cause mild to severe anaemia.
iv. Support therapy in the form of i.v. electrolyte/amino acids, blood transfusions, parenteral antibiotics and multivitamins and nursing. For *Plasmodium* sp.: chloroquine phosphate (12–15 mg kg^{-1} p.o. at 0, 12, 24, 36 and 48 hours) in addition to primaquine (0.75–1 mg kg^{-1} p.o. once). Therapy for other blood parasites has not been recommended.

167 i. Visceral gout.
ii. Hypovitaminosis A, due to the failure of normal cell differentiation, which can cause keratinization of the kidneys, interfering with the excretion of urates. These urates can then deposit in soft tissue and joints.
iii. It is frequently concluded that excessive levels of protein in the diet cause gout. This is based on the logic that protein contains nitrogen, which leads to the synthesis of uric acid in the excretion of this excess nitrogen. High levels of protein in the diet have been correlated with high blood urate levels but such levels do not correlate with gout. The only nutritional deficiency that causes gout – except remarkably high levels of protein in chickens selected to get gout – is a vitamin A deficiency.
iv. Gout can also be a sign of almost any kidney disease. The underlying cause of the kidney damage must be determined, usually with the aid of histopathology.

168 Whenever your opinion is asked by the owner of an animal with regard to diagnosis or treatment performed by a colleague, you should inform this colleague that you have been requested by the owner to look into the case and ask to be sent all relevant information. In this case it is important to know that determination of plasma potassium concentration is problematic in birds since there is a time-dependent increase or decrease of plasma potassium concentrations depending on the storage conditions of uncentrifuged blood samples.

For example, when uncentrifuged, heparinized ostrich blood is stored for 1 hour at 0°C (32°F) there is a 20% increase in plasma potassium concentration, but when the same blood is stored at 20°C (68°F) there is a 10% decrease in 1 hour. In pigeons, plasma potassium concentrations decline rapidly when blood is stored at room temperature. After 10 minutes the reduction was 10% and declined by 65% after 120 minutes. It should be ruled out therefore that the high plasma potassium concentration is not caused by an artefact.

Although hypoadrenocorticism is a well-known cause for electrolyte disturbances in mammals, Addison's disease has hitherto not been reported in parrots. Before life-long treatment is prescribed, it should be verified that the correct diagnosis is made. Occasionally erroneous conclusions are made with regard to adrenocortical function in birds because the same glucocorticoid assay is used as the one used in dogs. However, the major glucocorticoid in birds is corticosteron and not cortisol, as in dogs. In the ACTH stimulation test, therefore, plasma corticosteron concentrations before and after stimulation with ACTH should be determined.

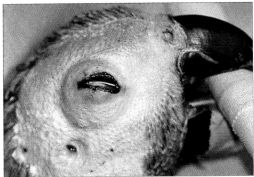

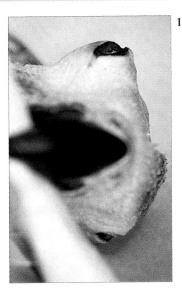

169 This 12-year-old, male African grey parrot (169a, b) has a retrobulbar mass diagnosed using ultrasound. It has been decided that the eye must be enucleated to gain access to the mass. Describe the procedure for enucleation in birds and how it differs from the same procedure in mammals.

170 Eversion of the cloaca (170) should be included as part of any psittacine physical examination. Why?

- To determine the sex?
- To examine the cloacal mucosa for any cloacal papillomas?
- To diagnose cloacal prolapse?
- To check mucosal colour to detect anaemia?

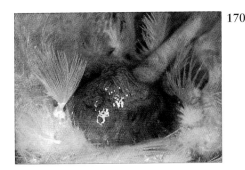

171 A clinically normal appearing channel-billed toucan (*Ramphastos vitellinus*) is diagnosed with iron storage disease (171).
i. What are the treatment options you can offer this concerned owner?
ii. Is the condition considered curable in toucans?

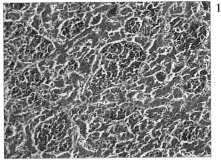

169 Birds have a very short optic nerve so excessive traction on the globe can result in damage to the optic chiasma and the contralateral optic nerve rendering the contralateral eye blind. It is also possible that the brain could be adversely affected by excessive traction. Many birds have bone within the sclera – scleral ossicles – which can inhibit removal of the globe. In an effort to achieve better visualization of the muscles and blood vessels surrounding the globe, the cornea is incised and the lens and vitreous extruded to allow the globe to be collapsed. It is important to remove the lacrimal tissue as well as the eyelid margins to eliminate glandular tissue and provide a cut surface for the eyelids to heal to each other. The eyelids may be sutured together first and the skin along the lid margins incised a few mm from the edges circumferentially. Dissection is continued subcutaneously to remove all of the palpebral conjunctiva. Muscle attachments are transected until the optic nerve and associated vessels are all that remain attaching the globe to the orbit.

Haemostatic clips are applied to the stalk blindly without applying significant traction to the globe. The optic stalk is then transected distal to the clips. An angled clip applier is preferred as it allows the clips to be applied with minimal traction on the globe. Remaining haemorrhage is controlled with bipolar radiosurgical forceps. The eyelids are then closed routinely. An ocular prosthesis may be used to prevent the sunken appearance characteristic of avian enucleation.

170 Cloacal papillomatosis can be detected by inserting a swab into the bird's cloaca and gently everting it to examine the mucosal tissue to the level of the proctodeum. Dilute acetic acid solutions can be used to increase visibility of the papillomas.

171 i. There are currently two potential treatment options that may be offered to a client with an affected bird.

The first method involves the use of periodic phlebotomies. Blood should be let at a rate of 1% of the bird's body weight – i.e. 10% of blood volume – weekly, continued for a period of a year; for example for a 380 g toucan this would be 3.8 ml weekly. Haematocrit should be monitored regularly. The progress and usefulness of the phlebotomies should be reassessed every 4–6 months. Phlebotomies are a method that is commonly used in humans, and may extend for periods lasting more than a year.

The second method for lowering a toucan's hepatic iron involves the use of the chelating agent deferoxamine (Desferol, Ciba). This chelating agent has had limited use but may show great potential with additional clinical trials. It has been used at the rate of 100 mg kg^{-1} injected subcutaneously at 24 hour intervals. Response and cessation of the therapy should be monitored by serial hepatic biopsies, possibly at 120 day intervals. More individuals need to be assessed to better evaluate this treatment modality.

ii. Current research and clinical experience would suggest that it is not curable, as it may potentially be an inherited trait in certain species of ramphastides, as is the case with humans. As the numbers and variety of avian species is rapidly diminishing, it behoves the concerned avian clinician to offer the above treatment modalities to clients with toucans of species known to be affected by iron storage disease.

172 This 14-year-old, female umbrella cockatoo presented with an acute onset of dyspnoea. On presentation the bird was recumbent on the bottom of the cage gasping for breath. In **172** the bird has been stabilized.

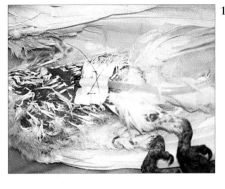

i. What procedure has been carried out to allow the bird to breathe again?
ii. When is this procedure indicated? After the bird was stabilized, you performed tracheal endoscopy and found three sunflower seeds in the trachea at the syrinx. You are able to see them but unable to retrieve them.
iii. Describe the approach for thoracic inlet tracheotomy used to retrieve the seeds.
iv. What are the potential postoperative complications?

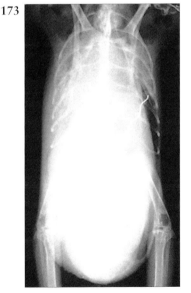

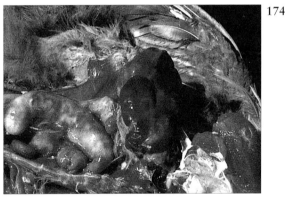

174 The abdominal contents found at post-mortem in an immature peafowl, which died acutely, are shown in **174**.
i. What is your diagnosis?
ii. Which species of bird is the condition particularly common in?
iii. What pathogen causes the disease?
iv. How does the victim become infected?
v. What prevention can be taken?
vi. Why is preventive medication on occasions ineffective?

173 This anorexic mynah bird (**173**) shows severe dyspnoea.
i. What abnormal findings are illustrated in this radiograph?
ii. What are the differential diagnoses?
iii. How would you confirm the diagnosis?

172 i. An air sac cannula has been placed to allow the bird to ventilate through the caudal thoracic or abdominal air sac.

ii. This procedure is primarily indicated to relieve respiratory distress associated with an upper airway obstruction; it does not generally help birds with primary lung disease. However, forced ventilation with oxygen through an air sac cannula may improve the arterial oxygen saturation.

iii. In order to best visualize the trachea and syrinx, the bird is positioned with the shoulders elevated at 50–60° allowing the surgeon to look down into the thoracic inlet. The syrinx cannot generally be retracted into the cervical region. The thoracic inlet approach to the distal trachea and syrinx is through a midline skin incision over the crop, which is carefully dissected for the overlying skin and reflected to the right to reveal the trachea dorsal to the ingluvies and oesophagus. Fat and the clavicular air sac must be dissected from the thoracic inlet to allow visualization of the trachea and associated structures. The sternotrachealis muscles are transected using radiosurgery to control haemorrhage. Stay sutures are placed through the trachea between rings and used to pull the syrinx into view. Alternatively, a hook can be inserted through the thoracic inlet to engage the syrinx and retract it into view.

A transverse tracheotomy is created several rings orad (towards the mouth) from the syrinx on the ventral aspect of the trachea through half of its diameter. Following removal of the seeds, the tracheotomy is closed with fine absorbable, monofilament material encompassing at least two rings on each side of the tracheotomy in a simple, interrupted pattern. Subcutaneous tissues and skin are closed routinely.

iv. Potential postoperative complications include subcutaneous emphysema, stricture and granuloma formation at the suture material. It is best to place knots external to the lumen of the trachea to minimize the chances for intraluminal granuloma formation.

173 i. There is generalized abdominal enlargement. A piece of metal wire is visible in the region of the left thoracic air sac, lung and abdomen.

ii. The bird may have ingested the wire, which may have caused peritonitis and ascites. Alternatively, the wire may be within the pectoral muscle and not within the abdomen. In the latter case the abdominal enlargement may indicate hepatomegaly and ascites due to haemochromatosis.

iii. All cases should be radiographed from two views at 90° angles to each other. A barium meal and/or ultrasound would confirm the liver size.

174 i. Blackhead.

ii. Turkeys and peafowl.

iii. *Histomonas meleagrides.*

iv. Young, non-immune birds ingest *Heterakis gallinae* worms which are infected with *H. meleagrides.*

v. Young birds may be fed a concentrate pellet containing dimetridazole.

vi. As most peafowl range freely, eating any garden morsels they can find, they often do not eat sufficient volumes of medicated feed to control the disease. The birds must be shut in daily for sufficient time to allow adequate medicine ingestion.

175 A three-week-old, hand-fed Moluccan cockatoo chick (*Cacatua moluccensis*) was presented with a three-day history of delayed emptying of the ingluvies. The chick weighed 186 g. An aspirate of the ingluvies was performed for cytological evaluation (**175**).
i. What cytodiagnosis do you make?
ii. What therapy would you recommend for this condition?
iii. What predisposing conditions lead to the development of this condition in hand-fed chicks?

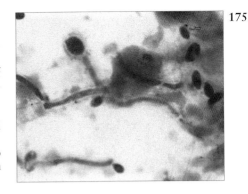

176 i. What is the condition and aetiology responsible for the ocular discharge in the right eye of this long-eared owl (*Asio otus*) (**176**). The condition is illustrated using mydriasis induced by air sac perfusion anaesthesia (APA).
ii. Which additional ophthalmological diagnostic procedures would you perform?
iii. What is the treatment?

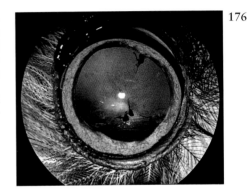

177 An adult, five-year-old male goose is presented (**177a**) with chronic progressive lameness. The bird has a half-acre yard (which is approx. 2024 m^2) and a plastic wading pool.
i. What are the relevant differential diagnoses?
ii. What treatment options are available?
iii. How could this condition be prevented?

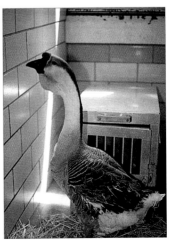

175 i. The Wright's-stained smear reveals many oval yeast and hyphae. There is no apparent inflammatory response. The yeast and hyphae are compatible with a severe yeast infection, most likely candidiasis, involving the ingluvies.

ii. An antifungal drug is indicated for the treatment of candidiasis. The presence of hyphae is suggestive of invasion of the mucosa by the yeast and the potential for a systemic infection. Therefore, a systemic antifungal – e.g. itraconazole at 10 mg kg^{-1} p.o. b.i.d. for 7 days – should be used along with a local or topical antifungal, e.g. nystatin 300 000 IU kg^{-1} p.o. b.i.d. or t.i.d. for 7–10 days.

iii. Immunosuppressive conditions and trauma to the ingluvies lead to the development of candidiasis. Predisposing factors include hypothermia, feeding a formula that is too cold or too hot, poor nutrition, antibiotic therapy and systemic illness from other causes.

176 i. This is post-traumatic subluxation of the lens with rupture of the lens capsule and zonula fibres in the ventronasal lens periphery with consecutive coloboma of the lens and iridodonesis. There is traumatic nuclear cataract and false cataract with multiple black pigment spots on the anterior lens capsule with slight dyscoria of the iris. There is a dim reddish fundus reflex due to the absence of a tapetum lucidum and the poorly pigmented fundus in nocturnal bird species.

ii. The slight dyscoria of the iris as well as the black spots on the anterior lens capsule are residues of the posterior surface of the iris due to partial dissolution of the posterior synechia. Measure the intraocular pressure immediately – physiological value 10.2 ± 2.1 mmHg – preferably using an electronic tonometer. This may initially be slightly decreased due to uveitis but may be increased by up to 40 mmHg, indicative of glaucoma. Since this is a condition with a traumatic aetiology, ophthalmoscopy of the contralateral eye – which usually appears outwardly healthy – is indicated for prompt recognition of intravitreal haemorrhage.

iii. Rupture of the lens capsule leads to lens protein leakage into the anterior chamber; upon contact with the anterior uvea this is recognized as foreign material, resulting in uveitis. Cataract resection – preferably by phacoemulsification – is obligatory to prevent complete inflammatory destruction of the eye.

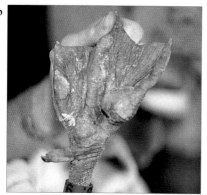

177b

177 i. Differentials would include trauma, osteoarthritis, skeletal tuberculosis, septic arthritis, mycoplasmal infection or pododermatitis. The diagnosis was a fibrogranulomatous lesion arising due to a foreign body penetration or due to chronic trauma of the plantar aspect of the foot (**177b**).

ii. Large plantar granulomas need to be surgically excised to relieve discomfort and lameness. Radiography is indicated in severe cases to exclude a secondary osteomyelitis; also deep debridement and bandaging for a minimum of 2 weeks.

iii. Prevention involves the provision of clean, atraumatic surfaces, i.e. no rough concrete, avoiding rocks and hard surfaces where possible together with free access to clean, deep water for swimming.

178 Inspect **178** for the gross post-mortem appearance of an avian embryo – a sandhill crane – that died during the last third of incubation.
i. What do you suspect as the cause of death?
ii. What is the likely aetiology of this condition?
iii. What are some appropriate measures one can take to prevent this problem?

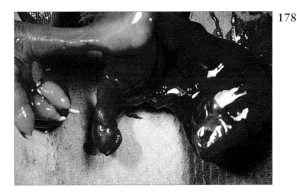

179 In **179** the veterinarian is placing a needle in the hock joint.
i. How effective is joint anaesthesia in ratites for identifying lameness sites?
ii. Name two diseases where joint anaesthesia may be a helpful identification aid in ostriches.

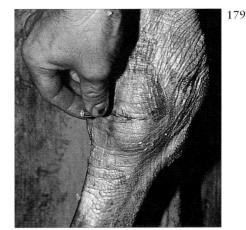

180 **i.** What is the problem in this young goose (**180**)?
ii. What is the cause?
iii. How is it best managed or prevented?

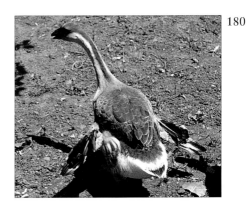

178–180: Answers

178 i. The embryo has consolidated yolk sac contents indicating an infection (omphalitis).

ii. Coagulated yolk material is often seen in bacterial infections associated with *Salmonella* sp. or *E. coli*. Both are associated with omphalitis and embryonic death occurring during the last third of incubation. Infections acquired during or immediately after laying or during incubation may result in mortality before or after hatching.

iii. Yolk sac contents should be cultured to obtain a positive identification of the organism involved. Infection may be associated with an infected female reproductive tract. Aviary dust settling on eggs is another source of infection – bacterial counts as high as 10^5–10^6 bacteria per g of dust have been found in aviary dust. Additionally, dirty pens, nests or unhygienic egg collection techniques are a possible source of infection. Parent birds may track faeces on to eggs, resulting in contamination. Therefore, reduction in faecal contamination and dust in the aviary and incubator are important. Fumigating or disinfecting eggs shortly after laying can reduce the risk of infection. A low incubation temperature has been shown to increase the incidence of *E. coli* infection. Regular candling during artificial incubation will reduce the risk of infection and contamination of other currently viable eggs by removal of non-viable eggs.

179 i. Joint anaesthesia is an excellent way to localize non-specific lameness of the leg in ratite species.

ii. Two diseases – where joint anaesthesia may be helpful – are osteochondrosis and cruciate ligament damage.

180 i. This condition known as 'slipped' or 'angel' wing involves an outward rotation of the carpal joint or the major metacarpal bone.

ii. Slipped wing is caused by the weight of the growing flight feathers placing an excessive force on the muscles and ligaments of the carpal area. The condition is most common in fast growing species such as geese which would normally feed by grazing on grass and other vegetation. It is more common in males and is always seen during the blood feather growth phase. Manganese and vitamin D_3 deficiencies have been implicated but genetics and in particular growth management have a greater role. If grazing birds – which typically eat grass having a crude protein content of 17–18% – are given a higher protein content grower pellet, such that they grow faster than they were designed to, the condition will occur.

iii. Treatment involves the application – preferably within 24–48 hours of occurrence – of a figure-of-eight bandage to bring the primaries back against the wing itself. Such a dressing, if combined with nutritional restriction, will result in a correction in 3–4 days. If a mature bird is presented with this abnormality, it may be corrected by cutting the major metacarpal and introducing a pin into the medulla. The lateral rotation along the length of the metacarpal is corrected and the bone allowed to heal, prior to pin removal.

181 i. Which condition is shown in the conjunctiva of the left eye of this Salvin's Amazon parrot (*Amazona autumnalis salvini*) (**181a**)?
ii. Which diagnostic procedure would you choose to make a definitive diagnosis and what are the differential diagnoses?
iii. Is there a treatment and what is the significance for any in-contact birds and the keeper?

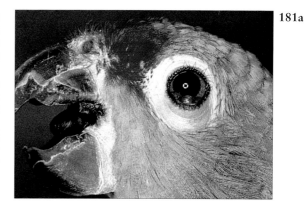

181a

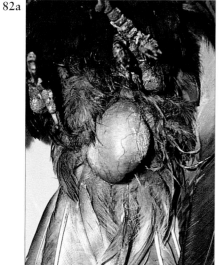

182a

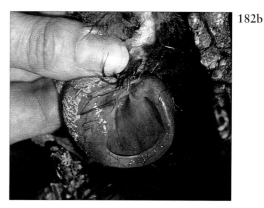

182b

182 A parrot breeder has found his Vasa parrot's cloacal region looking like this (**182a, b**) though the bird appears healthy. What is your advice?

181b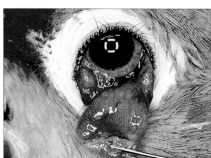

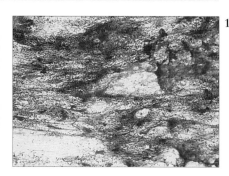 181c

181 i. Chemosis and granular conjunctivitis caused by a localized *Mycobacterium avium* infection.

ii. After everting the lower eyelid, the typical multiple subconjunctival granulomas become visible (**181b**). Diagnosis is made by taking a conjunctival biopsy – preferably under combined isoflurane and topical local anaesthetic – for a crush preparation for Ziehl–Neelsen staining. This specific stain directly identifies the Mycobacteria as acid-fast red rods (**181c**). Possible clinical differential diagnoses for this disease – which also occurs in other bird species – in particular pigeons, water fowl and predatory birds, are infections with *Pasturella multocida*, *Yersinia pseudotuberculosis*, *Staphylococcus aureus*, *Mycoplasma* sp., herpesvirus and poxvirus infections which may result in follicular conjunctivitis.

iii. There is no treatment: affected birds must always be euthanased. Examine contact birds serologically to demonstrate antibodies, haematology for a leucocytosis with a hypochromic microcytic anaemia and hyperfibrinogenaemia, and coproscopic tests for acid-fast bacilli of Mycobacteria (open tuberculosis) using enrichment methods (Sputofluol). Birds may be X-rayed to demonstrate possible tuberculous granulomas of other organs; hepatic endoscopy can be useful. Decontaminate aviaries using special tuberculocidal disinfectants. When localized, cutaneous tubercular lesions are found in birds; these are often caused by *Mycobacterium tuberculosis* infections, i.e. human pathogenic organisms. Although *M. avium* is zoonotic, *M. tuberculosis* is a much more serious human pathogen. It can certainly be passed from man to bird and possibly bird to man. It is essential to warn the handler of the zoonotic risk.

182c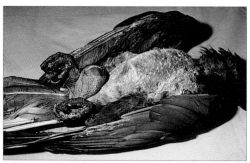

182 It is normal for the cloacal regions of the greater Vasa parrot (*Coracopis vasa*) and lesser Vasa parrot (*C. nigra*) to enlarge in the breeding season. A dead *C. vasa* has been plucked to show the cloaca (**182c**). This normal structure develops during the breeding season and will hang several cm below the body of the bird. This happens in both the male and the female; its function is unknown.

183 On entering a client's establishment, 183 is seen. What is your reaction? Why? The photograph shows a Harris hawk feeding from a freshly killed, ex-wild pigeon. List all disease risks associated with this practice and describe how, if possible, any of them may be minimized.

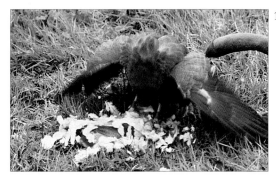

184 This anorexic Amazon parrot regurgitates and has undigested seeds in the faeces.
i. What abnormalities are on the X-ray (184)?
ii. What are the differential diagnoses?
iii. What clinical signs could be expected in a case of psittacine proventricular dilatation syndrome and what is the causative organism?

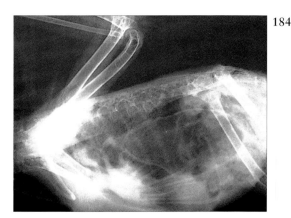

185 Changes in size and colour of the liver can be diagnosed during endoscopic examination (185). If abnormal findings are observed, liver biopsy is indicated.
i. What is the preferential approach for taking a liver biopsy?
ii. Does one have to pay special attention to haemostasis?

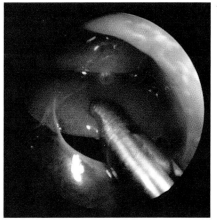

183 The feeding of pigeons may transmit or cause a number of diseases. The common infections or other disease risks are as follows. Infectious diseases:

- Newcastle disease (PMV1).
- Paramyxovirus (PMV1 pigeon) or PMV3.
- Falcon herpesvirus.
- Avipox.
- *Mycobacterium avium.*
- Salmonellosis.
- Trichomoniasis.

Poisonings:

- Lead.
- Alphachlorulose.
- Mercury.
- Pesticides, e.g. Fenthion; DDT.

Although pigeon carcasses are nutritionally beneficial to raptors, their ingestion is associated with a number of disease risks and hence pigeon should ideally not be fed to raptors at all. As trichomonads are temperature sensitive, the chilling or freezing of a carcass prior to thawing and feeding will greatly reduce the risk of this disease, although freezing has little effect on the risk of viral infections. Alternatively, where possible, one can medicate a pigeon population for trichomoniasis prior to the killing and feeding of the pigeons.

184 i. The proventriculus is severely distended, the wall is very thin and there is gas in the intestinal loops.
ii. Likely diseases – which lead to enlarged proventriculus and undigested seed in the faeces – are psittacine proventricular dilation syndrome (PPDS), heavy metal poisoning or any other cause of severe proventriculitis. The latter may be caused by bacterial agents such as *E. coli* or *Klebsiella* sp. or by *Candida* sp. infections. Severe infestations of nematodes or cestodes can lead to an enlarged proventriculus.
iii. Clinical signs often start with a change in the consistency, colour and composition of the faeces, which becomes very thin, intense green and may contain undigested seeds. The faeces of pellet-eating PPDS affected birds becomes voluminous and foetid and are usually pale brown. Most patients also exhibit signs of weakness, anorexia, depression and sometimes central nervous symptoms such as ataxia. Characteristic histological findings are of a lymphoplasmocytic infiltrate of the nervous tissue, detectable on proventricular or crop biopsy. The disease is segmental in nature. Biopsy tissue should include a blood vessel as the nerves proximate to these, so that the pathologist is more likely to examine a relevant section of tissue. The disease is thought to be of viral origin.

185 i. The preferred approach – for examination of the liver and the collection of liver biopsies – is via the ventral midline, immediately posterior to the sternum.
ii. Usually no special attention is needed for haemostasis when performing liver biopsy.

186 A radiograph of a 15-day-old Lugger falcon (*Falco jugger*) (186).
i. What abnormality is evident?
ii. How would it be treated?
iii. What soft tissue complication often presents with this condition?
iv. Apart from the abnormality shown, what other bony anatomical abnormalities are often seen as part of the same clinical situation?
v. What is the aetiology of the condition?
vi. In view of your previous answer, what common factor is often true of all affected chicks?
vii. What prophylactic measures would you recommend in order to prevent subsequent cases?

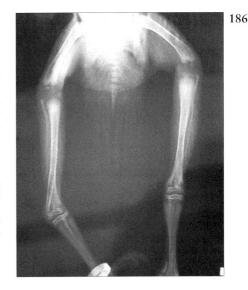

187 i. A Hawaiian goose or Ne-Ne (*Branta sandvicensis*), from a sizeable collection of mixed waterfowl, is shown in 187, with multiple white lesions in the liver. List the differential diagnoses in order of probability.
ii. How would you confirm your diagnosis?
iii. Does this disease have implications for the remainder of the collection?
iv. What factors affect the differential rates of infection in different species of waterfowl?

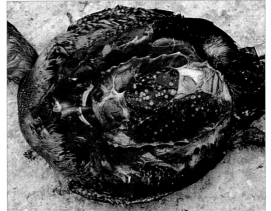

186 i. Varus of the distal tibiotarsus.

ii. Surgery should be performed to remove a strip of periosteum and growth plate from the inner curvature. The leg may then be realigned in a straight position and a cast applied for 14 days. When the cast is removed the leg should be straight and fully functional.

iii. Luxation of the calcaneal tendon.

iv. Tibial dyschrondroplasia, bowing in the mid section of the tibiotarsus, valgus or varus and rotation along the longitudinal axis of the tibiotarsus.

v. The condition is secondary to trauma to the growth area, although there is often a dietary imbalance of calcium to phosphorus (i.e. insufficient calcium in relation to the level of phosphorus). Alternatively, the contents of the egg itself, when laid, may have been deficient in calcium. Clinical incidence can be reduced by supplementation with $1\alpha,25$-dihydroxycholecalciferol and avoided by the ingestion by both parents and young of a balanced 'whole carcass' diet. Excessive growth rates can lead to problems even when a normally adequate diet has been supplied.

vi. All affected raptor chicks that were suffering from this condition (those examined by the contributor) have been second or third clutch chicks, where the first clutches have been pulled and the female recycled in a short period.

vii. It is suggested that any female raptor that is likely to recycle should receive a good diet with a suitable Ca:P ratio, together with a Ca and vitamin D_3 supplement.

187 i. The differential diagnoses are avian tuberculosis (*Mycobacterium avium*), pseudo-tuberculosis (*Yersinia* sp.) and lymphosarcoma.

ii. Either by impression smears of the affected tissue, stained with modified Ziehl–Neelsen, test for acid-fast bacilli, or by culture of the organism although this typically takes several weeks.

iii. The disease is highly contagious within a collection due to contamination of the ground by subclinical or preclinical cases, leading to subsequent ingestion of the organism and potential infection of unaffected birds.

iv. Infection is generally by the oral route, hence the method of feeding. Grazing, dabbling or diving will affect the potential level of ingestion of infected material whilst feeding. Those ducks feeding around the water margin – dabblers – will ingest the highest numbers of infective organisms. Furthermore, species being kept far from their climatic origin suffer stress as a consequence and hence show an increased incidence. Saltwater species kept on fresh water demonstrate an increased incidence. Certain species – e.g. white-winged wood duck (*Cairina scutulata*) and Hawaiian goose (*Branta sandvicensis*) – are more susceptible to infection, irrespective of the method of husbandry.

The rate of pathogenesis is variable between species. White-winged wood duck typically suffer rapid progress, dying within 2–4 months from the start of the infection, while some swans and geese will show no clinical signs of disease until 2–3 years from the start. However, during this period they may be faecal shedding continuously, leading to high levels of environmental contamination.

188 i. A mute swan (*Cygnus olor*) is radiographed, revealing a dilated oesophagus packed with radiolucent material. What are the likely causes?

A blood sample was taken from this swan, and the results are shown below:

Parameter	Results	Normal range
Hb	68 g l⁻¹ (6.8 g dl⁻¹)	110–165 g l⁻¹ (11–16.5 g dl⁻¹)
MCHC	301 g l⁻¹ (30.1 g dl⁻¹)	290–365 g l⁻¹ (29–36.5 g dl⁻¹)
PCV	26%	32–50%
TP	36 g l⁻¹ (3.6 g dl⁻¹)	35.5–54.5 g l⁻¹ (3.55–5.45 g dl⁻¹)
Calcium	2.32 mmol l⁻¹ (9.28 mg dl⁻¹)	2.19–2.89 mmol l⁻¹ (8.76–11.56 mg dl⁻¹)
Uric acid	125 mmol l⁻¹ (2.10 mg dl⁻¹)	126–700 mmol l⁻¹ (2.12–11.77 mg dl⁻¹)
Glucose	10.5 mmol l⁻¹ (189 mg dl⁻¹)	6.2–12.6 mmol l⁻¹ (111.7–227 mg dl⁻¹)
Cholesterol	5.65 mmol l⁻¹ (218.5 mg dl⁻¹)	3.0–7.8 mmol l⁻¹ (116–301 mg dl⁻¹)

ii. Taking into account the radiograph and the blood results, what is your diagnosis?
iii. What other test could be carried out to check the diagnosis?
iv. What treatment would you give? Name two different drugs that could be used, and explain any differences in their action.
v. For how long would you maintain therapy?

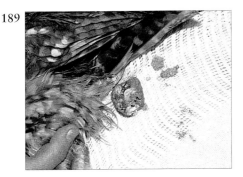

189 The tawny owl (**189**) was presented apparently weakened, straining frequently and passing only small volumes of faeces and uric acid.
i. What condition was this bird suffering from?
ii. What is the recommended treatment?
iii. When does the condition most often arise?
iv. List three other causes of abdominal straining.

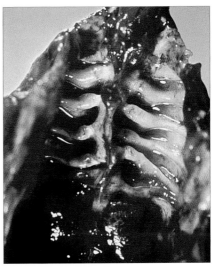

190 i. What condition is shown in **190**?
ii. What role might chronic egg laying play in this condition?
iii. What level of calcium in the diet might prevent this?
iv. What progression of eggshell quality changes occur as a hen lays eggs when fed a calcium-deficient diet?

188 i. These findings are consistent with oesophageal dilation due to 'proventricular dilation syndrome' (although not previously reported in swans, it has been diagnosed in Canada geese), an oesophagus impacted with long-stem grass – which is seen on occasion when swans or geese graze on long-stem grass – or oesophageal dilation due to heavy metal poisoning with secondary vegetable matter impaction.
ii. Acute lead poisoning.
iii. Blood lead analysis (or liver/kidney biopsy) or ALAD activity.
iv. CaEDTA is the traditional therapy – 35 mg kg^{-1} b.i.d. i.v. or i.m. as a chelation agent – acting on circulating blood lead, although it can be nephrotoxic. D-penicillamine may also be used – 55 mg kg^{-1} b.i.d. p.o. – and is said to chelate lead not only in the circulation but also in soft tissues such as liver and kidney. DMSA – 25–35 mg kg^{-1} b.i.d. p.o. 5 days per week for 3–5 weeks – is a water-soluble chelating agent shown to be effective in birds, but not nephrotoxic.
v. Previously, therapy has been given until clinical signs regress after 5 days to 4 weeks. However, there is good evidence of cases of rebound toxicosis from bone lead reserves as they re-enter the blood system, hence therapy in chronic cases, such as this, should continue for 2 weeks after the total recovery from clinical signs. The swan should be monitored further after this time.

189 i. The owl had a cloacal urolith.
ii. Once diagnosed the urolith may be broken up inside the cloaca with a pair of forceps and removed piecemeal. A certain amount of local trauma is likely to be caused, hence prophylactic antibiotics should be administered for 3–5 days following removal.
iii. The condition arises most often in breeding birds during or following incubation of their eggs. Some birds sit very tight, failing to get off the eggs and void their cloacal contents at irregular intervals. Precipitation of urates in the cloaca can, in time, lead to the formation of a uric acid concretion: a urolith.
iv. Three other causes of abdominal straining are:

• Enteritis, which, if severe, can lead to intersusception followed by colonic prolapse.
• Egg binding.
• Oviductitis, which can lead to a prolapsed oviduct.

190 i. Rickets of the ribs.
ii. Chronic egg laying on a calcium-deficient diet results in bone thinning in cockatiels. This leads to bone fractures that are difficult to treat due to the fragile bone structure of the depleted bird. Handling fragile birds may lead to iatrogenic fractures.
iii. The level of calcium that allows cockatiels to lay eggs at a sustained rate is a 0.4% diet. If no other treatment is given to chronic layers, a level of 0.4% calcium in the diet is essential to maintain bone strength.
iv. Cockatiels have the capacity to store enough calcium in their bones to produce two to four eggs of normal shell thickness before a calcium-deficient diet begins to cause eggshell thinning. As more eggs are laid, shells become thinner until egg laying ceases or shell-less eggs are produced.

191 This nine-year-old female hybrid macaw (191) presented for treatment of the mass protruding from its vent. The mass had been removed approximately a year earlier and the base cauterized with silver nitrate. Now the mass has recurred and the bird strains and vocalizes when voiding urine and faeces. On physical examination the mass appears to arise from the cloaca and is circumferential.

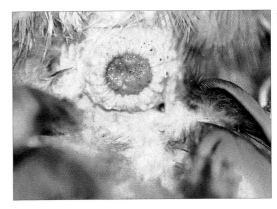

i. What is the most likely diagnosis?
ii. What surgical treatment options might be offered?
iii. What is the aetiology?
iv. What malignant neoplasia has been associated with this condition in Amazon parrots?
v. What is the long-term prognosis for curing this tumour?

192 A two-week-old duckling is presented for increased open-mouthed breathing and lethargy (192a).
i. What additional history would be helpful in order to make a preliminary diagnosis?
ii. The chick is very dyspnoeic and easily distressed. What are the best options in order to confirm the diagnosis?
iii. How would you treat and prevent this problem?

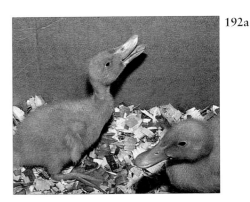

193 There are several situations where intubation of an air sac may be advantageous. These include airway obstructions and procedures such as surgery or diagnostic tests involving the upper airway and surgery of the oral pharynx, where intubation of the glottis may interfere with the procedure. Where is the most common location for air sac intubation?

• The cervicocephalic air sac.
• The clavicular air sac.
• The anterior air sac.
• The abdominal air sac.

191–193: Answers

191 i. Cloacal papilloma, though histology would be required to confirm the diagnosis.
ii. Various methods for surgical removal of these masses have been employed including cold blade excision, application of caustic substances, radiosurgical excision, cryosurgical removal and laser surgery. None of these methods has been consistently successful and recurrence is common.
iii. A viral aetiology has been proposed and may be most likely. In light of this, some emphasis has been placed on the development of autogenous vaccines as an adjunct to surgical therapy. These vaccines have failed consistently to control tumour regrowth. Some have indicated that chronic cloacal infection may predispose to the development of cloacal papillomas, and culture for organisms such as *E. coli* may be indicated.
iv. Bile duct carcinoma has been associated with cloacal papillomas in Amazon parrots. This lends support to the theory of a viral aetiology as some viruses are capable of inducing malignant transformations.
v. The prognosis for curing the problem is guarded to poor. Recurrence is common. Internal papillomas – oropharyngeal; proventricular; ventricular – are often fatal.

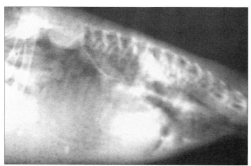

192 i. How many other ducklings are affected and what sort of brooder and rearer equipment is used?
ii. Since the bird easily stresses, oxygen was administered prior to slow induction with isoflurane anaesthetic to enable a tracheal examination and radiography. Placement of an abdominal air sac tube will often relieve dyspnoea.
iii. A radiograph (192b) revealed pulmonary densities that were suggestive of aspergillous lesions. Brooder pneumonia is caused by humid, cramped conditions with suboptimal ventilation. Treatment involves the setting of only clean eggs, the cleansing of eggshells prior to incubation, e.g. by UV light, together with improved brooder conditions and the administration of antifungal agents, such as itraconazole, to affected birds. Prognosis for affected young ducklings is poor.

193 The tube is most often placed into the left abdominal air sac because of its relatively greater size although the right abdominal and cervical air sacs may be used. The bird is positioned in dorsal or right lateral recumbency and the location for the tube is chosen so that it will not interfere with, or be occluded by, the legs if the tube is to be left in place in the conscious bird. Most often the tube is placed just lateral to the ventriculus and medial to the thigh. This will place the tip of the tube in the left abdominal air sac. If the situation permits, the area is prepared for sterile surgery and a small skin incision is made at the location of the tube placement. Haemostats or blunt scissors are used to dissect through the body wall. A visual inspection is made of the area deep to the incision to ensure there is a clear area for the placement of the tube and a sterile shortened endotracheal tube or modified soft rubber feeding tube is inserted through the hole and the tube checked for patency. A 'butterfly' of tape is placed on the tube and sutures placed to attach the tube to the body wall. The tube may now be attached to the anaesthesia machine or left for the patient to breathe room air.

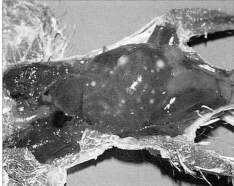

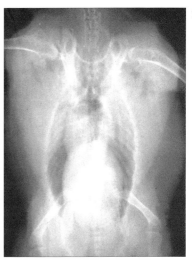

194 You are confronted with a flock of canaries with ruffling of the feathers, debilitation and high mortality. At necropsy, a dark, swollen, congested liver and spleen with small, yellow, focal granulomas are found (194).
i. What is your most likely presumptive diagnosis?
ii. How can you confirm this diagnosis?
iii. What should be your therapy?

195 i. What is abnormal on the radiograph (195)?
ii. What is your diagnosis and which species are especially prone to this condition?
iii. What are the causes of this condition and how can they best be controlled?

196 Five adult budgerigars (*Melopsittacu undulatus*) of varying ages and three juveniles (fledgelings) from a large aviary were presented with a history of regurgitation and weight loss. The aviary was experiencing a disease outbreak characterized by a sudden onset, high morbidity and low mortality. The eight birds were submitted for diagnostic evaluation of the flock problem. The affected birds exhibited evidence of regurgitation with accumulation of regurgitated material on the feathers surrounding the mouth and on the head. A crop aspirate for cytological evaluation was performed on all eight birds; the cytological findings were identical (196).
i. What is the cytodiagnosis?
ii. What is the treatment for this condition?

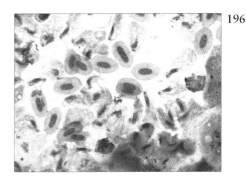

194 i. Infection with *Yersinia pseudotuberculosis* or *Salmonella typhimurium* is regularly seen in canaries during the winter months in birds of all ages. The clinical signs are not specific: in addition to those mentioned above, an acute catarrhal pneumonia and a typhlitis may be present.

ii. Many rod-shaped bacteria are seen in impression smears from all the organs. The diagnosis is confirmed after culturing the micro-organisms.

iii. The mostly commonly effective antibiotics are trimethoprim (with or without sulpha), amoxicillin or enrofloxacin via the drinking water or soft food. Once sensitivity test results are obtained, the antibiotic may need to be changed. Cleaning and disinfection are essential to prevent a relapse after therapy has been completed.

A connection has been suggested between contamination of food supplies by rodents and yersiniosis; although serotypes are often similar between rodent and avian *Yersinia* sp., no definite link has ever been proven. It is also likely that infection may occur through contact between infected feral birds and captive birds. In view of this contact, and access by rodents to birds or their food supplies, control of these factors is necessary.

195 i. The bird shows a moderately enlarged liver and thickened abdominal walls.

ii. The bird is obese. Obesity can predispose to lipoma formation. Fatty liver infiltration may occur. Obesity most commonly occurs in budgerigars, cockatiels, rose-breasted cockatoos and Amazon parrots.

iii. Many owners feed excessive quantities of unsuitable food such as cake, biscuits and sweets; it may be difficult to persuade the owner to change the food supplied. Birds are often selective in their feeding, choosing seeds, such as sunflower, or peanuts exclusively. These fattening seeds may need to be removed from the diet; the bird should be changed to a pelleted food if possible. Careful monitoring of the food consumption during the transitional phase is necessary to ensure that sufficient food is being consumed – boredom often leads to excessive food consumption. Environmental enrichment should be used – increased activity or exercise may be of value. Generally, there is lack of knowledge on the essential nutrient requirements of many avian species. This leads to a poor composition of many avian diets, forcing the birds to consume more food, and hence calories, than is necessary in order to ingest adequate quantities of essential nutrients.

196 i. The smear is highly cellular and contains numerous pale blue-staining, piriform-shaped cells each with a prominent nucleus, eosinophilic flagella, eosinophilic undulating membrane and axostyle. The cells are indicative of Trichomonad protozoa and a cytodiagnosis of trichomoniasis.

ii. Nitroimidazole drugs such as metronidazole (10–30 mg kg^{-1} p.o. b.i.d. for 10 days), dimetridazole (1 × 5 ml measure per 3.8 litres (1 tsp per gallon) of drinking water for 7 days) and carnidazole (100–200 mg kg^{-1} p.o. once) are usually effective in the treatment of trichomoniasis. Treatment in the drinking water or food, a better route for budgerigars, is necessary for flock problems.

197 Shown here are the feet of two raptors that were both presented with acute onset swelling of a toe, with an outwardly similar clinical appearance.
i. State what the lesion is in each case.
ii. What is the recommended treatment for the bird in **197a**?
iii. What is the recommended treatment for the bird in **197b**?

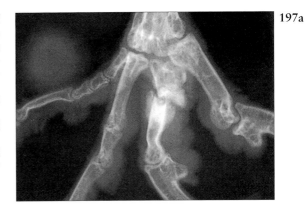

197a

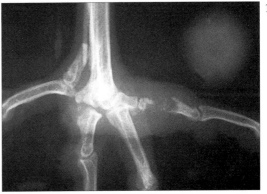

197b

198 i. List those medical causes of feather plucking (**198**) which are or may be infectious, contagious or transmissible.
ii. List the non-infectious medical, including metabolic, causes of feather plucking.
iii. Describe the diagnosis of the aetiologies described in i.
iv. List the environmental causes of feather plucking.
v. List the psychological causes of feather plucking.

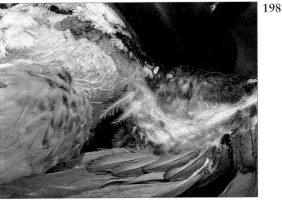

198

197 i. The bird in **197a** has suffered a fracture of digit 1; there is minimal soft tissue swelling.

The bird in **197b** has an acute, severe osteomyelitis affecting the lateral digit. The clinical history confirmed that the lesion had occurred following a cat bite to the toe 7 days previous. There is significant soft tissue swelling that has extended to the metatarsophalangeal joint (the ball of the foot).

ii. The bird with a fractured toe should be rested in the dark (to keep it quiet). A ball bandage encompassing the whole foot may be applied but must not be left on for more than 7 days. Any attempt to immobilize just the one toe will lead to disaster. If the whole foot is immobilized until the toe is fully healed, the flexor and extensor tendons may become involved in the bridging callous, preventing normal toe function in the future.

iii. The osteomyelitis affecting the bird in **197b** is clearly very lytic. In view of the tremendous lysis that has occurred in as little as 7 days, the future viability of the foot as a whole is at risk. In this situation, a decision was taken to immediately amputate that affected toe, effectively a damage limitation exercise. The infection was subsequently controlled and the foot saved, whereas it was believed that the toe was already well beyond help.

198 i. PBFD (circovirus); budgerigar fledgeling disease (*Polyomavirus*: French moult); ectoparasites (e.g. *Dermanyssus gallinae*); endoparasites (e.g. *Giardia* sp.); chlamydiosis; fungal dermatitis.

ii. Bacterial dermatitis; pulpitis or folliculitis; allergy; hepatitis; hypothyroidism; skin neoplasia; follicular cysts; post-traumatic injury, or arthritic or scar tissue pain; nutritional deficiency (e.g. hypovitaminosis A; B vitamin deficiencies; essential amino acid deficiencies (e.g. lysine)).

iii. PCR for PBFD and BFD; physical examination at day and night for ectoparasites; faecal examination for endoparasites; PCR/ELISA (antigen/antibody) for chlamydiosis; skin scrape microscopic examination and culture for fungal dermatitis; stained impression smear, culture and sensitivity for bacterial infections. Also, haematology and biochemistry, thyroid stimulation test, biopsy and histopathology, improved diet and monitoring response to therapy.

iv. Excess tobacco smoke; excessively dry atmosphere; excessive day length in direct sunlight; lack of environmental enrichment.

v. Attention seeking; boredom; overcrowding; environmental change or lack of routine; sexual frustration; excessive preening; post untidy feather or wing clipping.

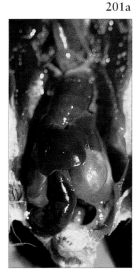

199 Most birds possess a uropygial gland or preen gland (**199**).
i. Where is it located?
ii. What does it produce?
iii. What are the main functions of its product?
iv. Name some birds that totally lack a preen gland.
v. What clinical abnormalities may affect the preen gland and how would each be treated?

200 Mention the three most likely causes of torticollis in pigeons and methods for prevention.

201a

201b

201 In small passerines, the small intestine may often be filled with blood (**201a**) or there may be a pale kidney with urate accumulation (**201b**) seen at necropsy.
i. What is the cause of the blood in the intestine?
ii. What is the most likely aetiology of the changes in the kidney?

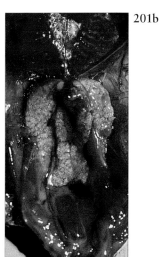

199 i. It is located on the dorsal surface of the rump, cranial to the point of attachment of the major tail feathers or rectrices.
ii. It secretes a rich oil of waxes, fatty acids, fat and water.
iii. When applied externally with the bill it cleans feathers and preserves feather moisture and flexibility, which assists in the durability and longevity of the feathers. Regular applications of the secretion to the plumage sustain its functions as an insulating and waterproofing layer. Water birds typically have large preen glands but whether the secretions of this organ are essential for keeping feathers dry and maintaining buoyancy remains to be verified.

The waxy secretion of the preen gland also helps to regulate the bacterial and fungal flora of feathers and skin. Finally, it has been suggested that components of the oil, when exposed to sunlight, become converted to activated vitamin D_3.
iv. Examples of birds that totally lack a preen gland are the ostrich, emu, cassowary and some doves, parrots and woodpeckers.
v. Obstruction of the preen gland duct (manual expression), neoplasia (surgery if possible), abscessation (debridement, culture and antibiosis), periuropygial dermatitis (control of self-trauma, antibiosis, anti-inflammatory agents and topical cleansing agents).

200 The three causes are *Salmonella typhimurium* var. *kopenhagen*, paramyxovirus infection and emtryl (dimetronidazole) toxicity.

Vaccination may be used to reduce the incidence of salmonellosis as well as totally preventing paramyxovirus. Inactivated vaccines are available for both diseases.

Dimetronidazole is used for the treatment of *Trichomonas* and *Hexamita* infections in pigeons. The advised dosage is 50 mg kg^{-1} per day. When it is given as a drinking water medication the dosage is 500 mg l^{-1} of drinking water. This assumes that each pigeon drinks 50 ml per day.

Be aware that during hot weather, or when the pigeons are feeding their young, water intake may be greatly increased and hence the dimetronidazole dosage may reach toxic levels. The first signs of intoxication are incoordination and circling; affected pigeons may even die. It is important to inform the owner regarding these complications.

201 i. The bleeding into the gut, often called 'haemorrhagic enteritis', is not enteritis in the true sense. This condition has been referred to by some previous workers as 'agonal bleeding'; it should be considered as a haemorrhagic diathesis. It is seen in small birds which for some reason ate nothing for over 24 hours, perhaps because they were too ill to eat – e.g. because of an infection or intoxication – or, more often, when they are fed the wrong food or no food at all, e.g. if the owner was away and someone else fed the birds. A typical concurrent finding is an empty stomach.
ii. A similar interpretation should be given to swollen, white kidneys, which are the result of uric acid precipitation in the collecting tubules; this occurs when birds do not drink. This condition is often falsely called renal gout but should not be interpreted as nephritis or gout. It should be differentiated from visceral gout based on impaired renal function or a high protein diet.

202 i. A wild Eurasian buzzard (*Buteo buteo*) was found beside a road, with a fracture. What are the initial considerations prior to the start of therapy?
ii. What essential factors must be ascertained at the time of examination?
iii. What are the essential differences between avian and mammalian bones, determining the methods of repair?
iv. What are the aims, in chronological order, when repairing an avian fracture?

203 A mitred conure (*Psitta-cara mitrata*) was presented with a 3 day history of weakness, lethargy and anorexia. The physical examination revealed a moderate reduction of the pectoral muscle mass and slight dyspnoea. The bird was weak, but able to perch. A blood profile revealed a mild to moderate leucocytosis at 18.6×10^9 l^{-1}, heterophilia at 17×10^9 l^{-1} and lymphopenia at 0.93×10^9 l^{-1}.

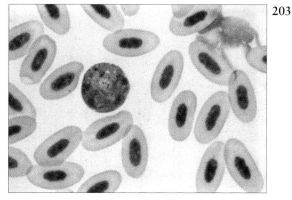

203

i. What is the cell demonstrated in the Wright's-stained peripheral blood film (203)?
ii. What is the significance of the cell demonstrated in the figure?

204 The liver in 204 is fatty.
i. What problems might occur with fatty liver?
ii. What nutritional factors are important in fatty liver?

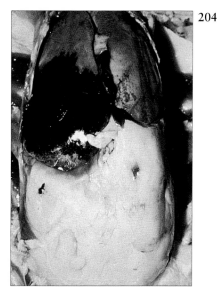

204

202 i. Since this is a wild bird, of a common species, the only aim should be to return it to the wild with full function to survive. Other significant damage to major or vital organs or structures should be assessed.

ii. The clinician must assess the following factors to determine if complete repair and return to normal function is possible. Which bone(s) is/are affected? Whether or not the fracture is simple, comminuted or open (compound). If open, how much contamination, devitalization or necrosis of the tissues is present? Is there any further significant soft tissue damage, in particular nerves, blood vessels or other essential structures such as the propytagium? How close is the fracture to a joint? After due consideration, decide whether the case is to be treated or euthanased.

iii. Avian bones have a thinner cortex and wider medulla, are more brittle and hence have a tendency to split or crack. Certain avian bones, such as the humerus are 'pneumatized' in order to minimize their weight. During preparation of the surgical site, care should be taken to prevent fluid from entering the air sac system. Stable, well-aligned avian fractures heal more quickly than mammalian bones.

iv. (1) Treat contaminated or infected wounds. (2) Preserve soft tissue, if necessary by applying splints or dressings. In view of the fragility of avian skin and the small soft tissue mass, special care is required to prevent desiccation. (3) Realign fractures or replace luxations. (4) Rigidly stabilize the fracture site, preventing any movement or rotation while, if possible, maintaining joint function and movement during healing. (5) Return the limb to full normal function with the aid of physiotherapy and controlled exercise.

203 i. The slide demonstrates a toxic heterophil. The heterophil shows increased cytoplasmic basophilia, abnormal cytoplasmic granules that include round, basophilic primary granules. This would be considered a 2+ to 3+ toxicity.

ii. Toxic changes in the heterophils represent the presence of a septicaemic or toxaemic condition, e.g. bacterial toxins. The greater the degree of toxicity and number of cells affected, the more severe the condition. Therefore, the presence of numerous heterophils showing signs of marked toxicity represents a severe condition and hence a poor prognosis for survival.

204 i. Fatty liver can lead to a number of pathologies. Such livers are often friable and haemorrhage from relatively mild traumas. As the level of fat increases, the level of liver function decreases until clinical signs are seen. Severe fatty liver can result in liver failure and death.

ii. Fatty liver can have a number of nutritional causes that all work through the same mechanism: inhibition of lipid transport. Modest levels of fat in the diet do not cause fatty liver in normal birds because this fat enters the bloodstream from the gut and is removed by adipose and other peripheral tissues. Fat stored in the liver is usually made there from a variety of precursors that are usually carbohydrates or their metabolites. Fatty liver occurs when the ability of the liver to make lipoproteins, the transport form of hepatic lipid, is impaired. This forces the liver to retain the fat that it manufactures. Two nutritional states that can inhibit this transport are protein malnutrition, which inhibits lipoprotein formation by limiting protein synthesis, and choline deficiency, which inhibits the linkage of protein to lipid in the synthesis of lipoprotein. The level of well-balanced protein in the treatment of fatty liver should be at least 12% with methionine and choline levels of 0.25–0.4% and 500–1300 mg kg^{-1} of diet respectively.

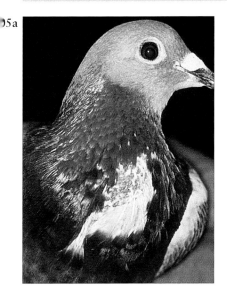

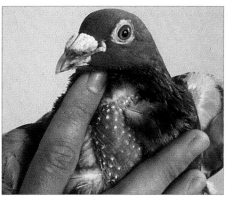

205 Racing pigeons with allopecia in the breast region are shown in 205a, b. What are the differential diagnoses of this condition? How can the condition be treated?

206 i. Describe the lesions in 206.
ii. What are the possible aetiologies?
iii. Which species are most commonly affected?
iv. What undesirable side-effect may be seen as a consequence of a bird's attempt to avoid the condition?
v. How can the condition be avoided?

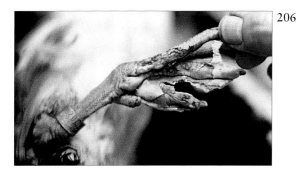

207 For which reason are these animals, racoons (207), important to aviculture?

• They often attack and kill birds in cages at night.
• They transmit sarcocystosis.
• They transmit rabies.
• They cause no problems.

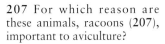

205 205a shows a pigeon with traumatic loss of feathers. The fractures of the feather shaft are thought to be caused by rubbing the breast on the sharp edges of the drinking pan. It is seen especially in nervous male pigeons who show aggressiveness towards other males trying to approach the drinking pans. This 'nervous behaviour' causes repeated friction of the throat area over the sharp edges of the drinking pans. Treatment of the condition is by pulling out the broken shafts after which the feathers will regrow in 3 weeks. At the same time, the number of drinking pans should be increased and the sharp edges covered with a plastic tube that has a longitudinal slit on one side. The level of the water in the pans should be raised.

205b shows a pigeon with parasitic loss of feathers. The parasite, *Cnemidocoptes laevis*, can be found in the feather follicle and the thickened base of the feather shaft, which is brushed with a scalpel blade on a microscopic slide for this purpose; other body areas may also be involved. Treatment with ivermectin is unsuccessful. After degreasing the plumage in a warm detergent solution, affected pigeons can be bathed in a 0.15% trichlorfon solution and left to dry in a warm environment; treatment can be repeated in 10 days. Infection of other pigeons occurs through direct contact; the environment is not thought to be a reservoir for reinfestation.

206 i. Dry gangrene and loss of tissue from the extremity of a duck's foot.
ii. Dry gangrene of extremities, as seen in mammals, has not been recorded in birds. This is caused by frostbite. Ergot poisoning has not been reported in birds.
iii. Waterfowl are most commonly affected by frostbite in this manner. Waterfowl lose heat by panting or heat exchange through their legs. However, most waterfowl are remarkably tolerant of frost effects, particularly if they have open water to swim in. When sedentary, they tend to squat down, sitting on their feet in order to maintain temperature. Species endogenous to warm climates, but kept in temperate areas, are most susceptible.
iv. Flamingos and other long-legged birds, being unable to sit on their feet to maintain heat, simply reduce peripheral circulation. Although they often avoid frostbite, the long-term effect of poor pedal circulation is a marked deterioration in dermal quality, leading to cracking and low-grade bacterial infections.
v. The condition is avoided by either not keeping warm climate birds in cold areas, or by keeping them inside during extreme weather. Even in such circumstances, water temperature may have to be artificially raised although water hygiene can be a problem if large numbers are housed together inside.

207 Racoons are an important predator of birds in outside aviaries. They hunt at night and can easily force entry into wire enclosures, often being undetected by the sleeping aviculturalist. Racoons are omnivores and enter the enclosure in search of food but will also attack sleeping birds, pulling them through the cage wire, often pulling off their heads and legs.

208 A three-year-old, male, yellow-naped Amazon parrot is presented to you with the complaint of being fluffed, sleepy and falling off its perch. Physical examination reveals the bird to be in good flesh, 7% to 10% dehydrated and uncoordinated. The bird's droppings are polyuric and red-brown in colour (208). Which is the most likely diagnosis in this case? Is it:

- Sarcocystosis.
- White muscle disease (hypovitaminosis E/selenium deficiency).
- Psittacosis (chlamydiosis).
- Plumbism (lead poisoning).

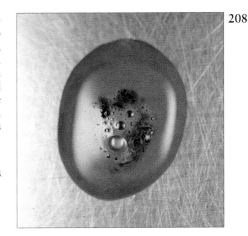

208

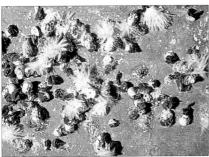

09a

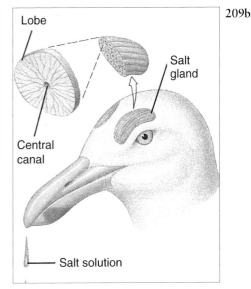

209b

209 Excretion of water and nitrogenous wastes by birds (209a) combines processes of the kidneys and the intestines and, in some species, the action of salt secreting glands (209b).
i. Do you see any advantage of urine mixing with faeces in the lower intestine?
ii. What is the advantage of excretion of nitrogen wastes in the form of uric acid, in birds, above excretion of nitrogen as urea in mammals?

208 Lead is a systemic, heavy metal poison that adversely affects every body system to which it is distributed. Abnormalities and clinical signs may vary with species, dose and duration of exposure. Signs may be vague and non-specific causing lead poisoning to be added to many lists of differential diagnoses. Neurologic, haematopoietic, GI, renal and immunological systems are most often involved. Central and peripheral nervous system signs include dull or poorly responsive mentation, wing droop, incoordination, muscle twitches and seizures. CNS signs are the result of perivascular oedema, increase in cerebrospinal fluid, necrosis of nerves and changes in neuronal metabolism. Peripheral neuropathy results from competition for calcium at neuronal junctions acutely and in more chronic cases leading to demyelination. Many of the clinical signs and laboratory findings result from lead damage to RBCs leading to premature destruction. The anaemia, polychromasia and anisocytosis is secondary to disruption of the formation of haem. The premature destruction of RBCs results in biliverdinuria (yellow-green to green-black coloration of urine and urate). In Amazon parrots, and occasionally other species, there will be haemoglobinuria which presents as a classic chocolate milk-to-blood-coloured dropping. With or without CNS signs, lead should be suspected in these patients. Many birds with lead toxicity are polyuric. This results from renal tubular damage caused by both the lead and haemoglobin. GI signs include anorexia, regurgitation and GI stasis or ileus including proventricular dilatation. GI signs are the result of both local effects of the lead on the GI tract and neurological pathology.

209 i. Avian kidneys differ in structure and function from those of reptiles or mammals. Urine produced by the kidneys mixes with faecal components in the lower intestine where additional water can be reabsorbed as needed.
ii. The most conspicuous physiologic adaptation for promoting water economy in birds is the excretion of nitrogenous wastes in the form of uric acid. The white crystals are synthesized in the liver and give bird droppings their characteristic colour; 90% of its secretion is via tubular secretion from reptilian-type nephrons and therefore largely independent of urine flow. Excretion of nitrogen as urea, in mammals, in aqueous solution requires flushing by large quantities of water but uric acid can be excreted as a semi-solid suspension – a colloidal solution – in which each molecule of uric acid contains twice as much nitrogen as a molecule of urea. Therefore birds require only 0.5–1.0 ml of water to excrete 370 ml of nitrogen as uric acid, whereas mammals require 20 ml of water to excrete the same amount of nitrogen as urea. Birds concentrate uric acid to amazing levels in the cloaca, just prior to defecation. It can be up to 3000 times the uric acid level in their blood.

210 Feather with stress bars (210). What is the cause of this feather lesion?

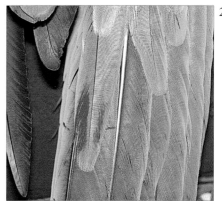

210

211 A blue-fronted Amazon parrot, about 20 years old, shows slight respiratory distress. The bird's neck appears swollen after falling from a table (211).
i. What radiographic abnormalities can be seen?
ii. What is your diagnosis?
iii. How would you treat the bird and what is the prognosis?

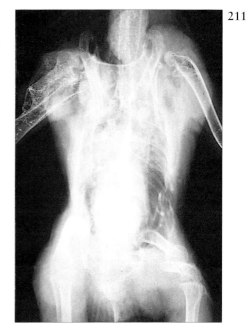

211

212 What are the three selection procedures which should be applied to a pigeon loft and why are they important.

210 'Stress marks', 'fret marks', 'segmental feather dystrophy' or 'hunger traces' are all terms for the same condition. This condition is caused by periods of stress during the development of the feather. Any stress – such as starvation, poor nutrition, environmental changes, dehydration, infection, chilling, over-heating, changes to new homes or cages – will cause the release of endogenous corticosteroids. Such lesions can be caused experimentally by the administration of glucocorticosteroids during feather development. Emotional stress is often such a factor. New owners, emotional turmoil in the home (owners going through a divorce, deaths in the family, etc.), new babies and new pets are a few common examples or factors that can cause emotional stress.

211 i. The radiographic abnormalities are: (1) old fractures of the left humerus and right femur; (2) distortion of the ribs and pelvis; (3) cervical emphysema.
ii. The healed multiple fractures and bone distortions are indicative of a historic metabolic bone disease: Ca/P/vitamin D_3 imbalance. This must have arisen when the bird was a chick. Deficiencies in Ca or D_3 or excesses of phosphorus will lead to such a condition as Ca absorption is dependent on the presence of vitamin D_3. Precursors of vitamin D_3 are converted to activated D_3 by exposure to UV light. Many psittacines are bred in the absence of direct sun exposure and may not receive sufficient UV light. High serum phosphorus levels can interfere with blood calcium levels causing a secondary hyperparathyroidism. The subcutaneous emphysema is probably caused by hyper-inflation of the cervical air sac. This may occur following trauma.
iii. The hyperinflation of the cervical air sac is corrected by making an incision over the swelling and allowing the air to escape. This incision must remain patent for at least 7 days to allow healing of the air sac wall internally. In non-refractory cases, the procedure may need to be repeated. Stents have been used for this purpose.

212 (1) It is necessary for the fancier to select those birds which he feels have the greatest potential to race well during that season, this selection being carried out in the first 2–3 months of the birds' lives, without fail. It is necessary to breed enough birds in order to facilitate selection, though some fanciers make the mistake of trying to race all youngsters of the season; the fancier should select to keep only 70–75% of pigeons bred in any year. Strict selection criteria must be followed. High quality pigeons develop more rapidly. Development of feather quality, skeletal structure and intelligence can be assessed; intelligence is indicated by a squab's ability to wean. Quality pigeons become territorial and are strong and viable; this quality is also important for the pigeon in the racing basket. A weak pigeon is more susceptible to stress, leading to ill health. Such birds should be removed from the loft, especially those with respiratory disease. Pigeons culled because of ill health should be examined to establish if loft treatment is necessary. Strict and early selection is one of the best preventive measures the fancier can make in disease control and loft quality improvement. (2) During the racing season, prior to each race, the fancier should select which of the available pigeons will be flown. Chosen pigeons should be healthy and in the best physical condition to perform optimally. The fancier should not use more than 40–50% of the available pigeons per race. The majority of the pigeons are 'losers'. These losers will lower the price percentage and they increase the risk of disease problems within the loft. (3) Another selection is for suitable breeding stock. This decision should be based on racing performance and disease resistance. A bird's racing ability is to a great extent determined by its genetic background. This ability may not necessarily be passed on to its progeny.

213 Two imported aracaris were presented for post-mortem examination (**213**). They had been in the aviculturalists collection for three and four years respectively. Both birds had seemed clinically normal, although they were slightly underweight. They were from different flights and were found dead within 3 hours of each other.

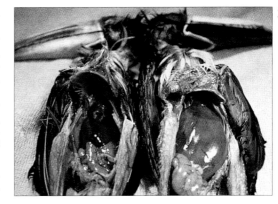

i. What are the two main disease conditions which should be considered in these two birds?
ii. How would one arrive at a final diagnosis?
iii. Are these two potential conditions contagious or infectious to the rest of the collection?

214 A two-year-old female hyacinth macaw, housed with a two-year-old male, had recently been moved into a new cage made out of galvanised wire (**214**). The pair had been chewing on the cage, and had popped many welds. She had developed loose, voluminous, malodorous, brilliant lime green droppings. She was anorexic, had lost weight and had developed pu/pd. Radiographs were negative for wire densities. Blood lead levels were normal. How should you proceed with the treatment?

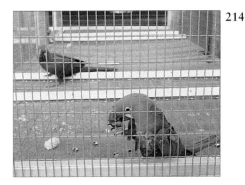

215 A falconer presents his red-tailed hawk (*Buteo jamaicensis*) for a routine 'well-bird' check up. Diagnostic assessment includes a haematology and chemistry profile. Your technician finds this strange object (**215**) in the stained blood film and asks you to take a look at it.
i. What is the object?
ii. What is the source?
iii. What do you tell your client about the clinical implications of this finding?

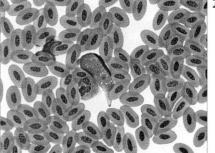

213 i. Both birds demonstrate extreme hepatomegaly. The two most frequently occurring disease conditions affecting toucans with this history – and with the gross clinical finding of extreme hepatomegaly – are avian tuberculosis and haemochromatosis. In all these conditions, toucans can be apparently clinically healthy and yet found dead shortly afterwards.

ii. A final diagnosis is determined following submission of tissues for histopathological examination. Findings of acid-fast organisms would be indicative of mycobacteriosis while special stains, in addition to disruption of normal hepatic architecture and replacement with iron, would be diagnostic for haemochromatosis.

iii. Avian tuberculosis is considered to be both infectious and contagious to a number of animal species, including humans, and some other mammal and avian species. Haemochromatosis, in contrast, appears to be due to some possibly inherited abnormalities in the bird's ability to metabolize iron and is not contagious or infectious

214 'New wire disease' can be seen when galvanised wire is used in the manufacture of cages and has not been treated properly: brushed with a wire brush and vinegar, cleaned with soapy water and then set out to dry prior to the placement of birds in the cage. Traces of lead and considerable quantities of zinc are found in this type of wire.

The pancreas, liver, kidneys, reproductive and gastrointestinal tracts are all affected by zinc. Necrotising ventriculitis is a common sequelae of zinc intoxication and may result in koilin exfoliation, intestinal obstruction and death. Zinc may cause ileus, gastroenteritis and dilated intestinal loops.

DMSA is now recommended for the treatment of lead and zinc poisoning in birds. DMSA is safe, is not nephrotoxic (which CaEDTA may be) and has been shown to decrease serum zinc concentrations experimentally in pigeons. The dosage of DMSA is 30 mg kg^{-1} p.o. b.i.d. for 10 days or 5 days per week for 3–5 weeks. Laxatives should be given to help mechanically remove any remaining metallic particles in the gut. Supportive care including rehydration, antibiosis, antifungals, gavage feeding and any other treatment based on additional diagnostic findings should be administered. If the patient is stable, surgery to remove radiographically visible metal densities can be attempted, or endoscopy or ventricular lavage may be used to remove metal particles. If particles still remain in the ventriculus, lavage is generally the easiest, quickest and least traumatic method of removal. For ingested galvanised wire, a neodymium–ferro–barium alloy magnet attached to a small diameter catheter may be used to retrieve metal from the GI tract. The cage mate should also be checked for plumbism and zinc toxicosis.

215 i. This is a *Leucocytozon* sp., a blood parasite affecting leucocytes and probably erythrocytes.

ii. Simulid – biting – flies are the common source of *Leucocytozoa* sp.

iii. Leucocytozoan infection is common in a variety of raptorial species but clinical disease due to a leucocytozoan is uncommon. Pyrimethamine has been suggested as a treatment.

216 An adult cockatiel presented with a history of lethargy. The previous year a mild hyperuricaemia was noted at another veterinary hospital. The diet was primarily a commercial formulated crumble. Another blood profile was submitted. The clinician noted leucocytosis and the following uric acid result:

Uric acid 1136 mmol l^{-1} (19.1 mg dl^{-1})) (normal range 136.8–583.6 mmol l^{-1} (2.3–9.8 mg dl^{-1}))

i. What is your differential result for the chemistry results?
ii. What is your treatment?
iii. What is the prognosis?

217 Shown in **217** is a set of magnification head loupes. What are the advantages of this type of loupe compared with hobby loupes, which are significantly less expensive?

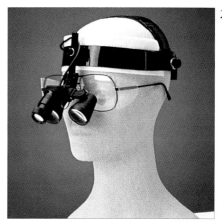

217

218 This double yellow-headed Amazon parrot (**218**) was bitten by a dog approximately an hour ago. What should your greatest concern be?

- Infection leading to sepsis.
- Damage to muscle leading to loss of wing function.
- Damage to tendons leading to loss of wing function.
- Exposure of tissue leading to hypothermia and dehydration.

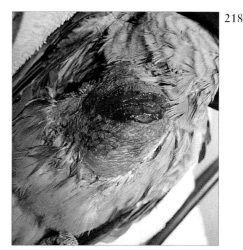

218

216 i. Differential diagnosis would include:

- Pre-renal dehydration (though result is rather high to be explained by this alone).
- Hypervitaminosis D.
- Toxic nephropathy.
- Soft-tissue gout.
- Bacterial nephritis.

Formulated diets have occasionally been associated with renal disease in cockatiels, although pu/pd is a typical presenting sign in such cases. Further diagnostics would include radiography, urinalysis and renal biopsy.

ii. Modification of the diet may ameliorate the change; in some cases treatment with allopurinol and/or colchicine is helpful.

iii. It is difficult to prognosticate birds based on uric acid results alone as this analyte is a relatively insensitive indicator of renal function. Marked elevation frequently occurs very late in the disease.

217 With this system, the surgeon is able to look around and bypass the lenses when they are not required, such as during surgical preparation. Hobby loupes cover the entire visual field.

The focal distance is ergonomically correct so the surgeon may sit upright with the back straight. With hobby loupes, the stronger the lens the shorter the focal distance, such that when using a 5× lens the surgeon's face must be only a few cm from the surgical field.

The lenses provide a focal range rather than a set focal distance. With hobby loupes, only objects that are the focal distance from the lenses are in focus. With surgical loupes everything within the focal range of several cm is in focus, allowing the surgeon more flexibility and an ability to visualize structures in more than one plane.

218 Infection. Bite wounds very often lead to a fatal septicaemia if not treated aggressively. The patient should be evaluated for its overall condition and treated appropriately for blood loss or hypotension. The extent of wounds should be evaluated. If the patient's condition allows, wounds should be thoroughly flushed and fractures stabilized. Aggressive antibiotics should be started early in the treatment. Piperacillin or cefotaxime combined with amikacin or tobramycin are a good choice and should be continued for up to 14 days. If septicaemia is suspected, treatment for septic shock should be instituted, i.e. intravenous fluids, rapidly acting steroids and intravenous bactericidal antibiotics.

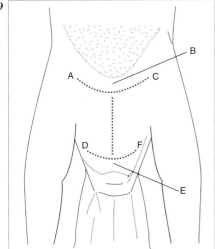

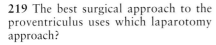

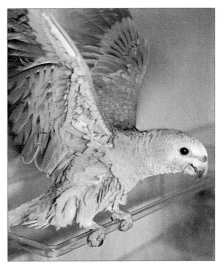

219 The best surgical approach to the proventriculus uses which laparotomy approach?

- ABC (transabdominal).
- BE (midline abdominal).
- CBEF (left abdominal flap).
- ABED and CBEF (double abdominal flap).
- Left lateral laparotomy between the last and the penultimate rib.

220 A six-month-old, hand-reared, orange-winged Amazon parrot (*Amazona amazonica*) is presented depressed (**220**). It has biliverdinuria, an elevated WBC (44.5×10^9 l^{-1}), an elevated Alk. Phos., SGOT and Bile Acids. An IFA titre and a DNA PCR faecal swab were both positive for chlamydiosis. What is the best treatment regime for this single pet bird?

221 Water intake in hatching altrichal birds (**221**) is regulated by the parent or surrogate parent.
i. How is water intake regulated by parents in growing birds?
ii. What are the effects of excessive water intake in growing cockatiels?

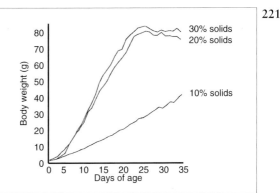

219 The last choice. The left lateral approach offers the greatest exposure and access to the proventriculus and is the least traumatic to the bird. The approach can be made from behind the last rib or between the last and penultimate ribs. Entry and closure can be accomplished rapidly, reducing anaesthetic and surgical time.

220 Doxycycline is the drug of choice for the treatment of chlamydiosis (in the USA). Enrofloxacin appears to be equally effective and is widely used in Europe. Using doxycycline, blood levels should be kept at 1 µg ml^{-1} for most of the dosage interval for successful treatment of chlamydiosis. Several dosage regimes are published using a variety of doxycycline preparations, both oral and injectable.

Oral doses of doxycycline should be administered at 25–50 mg kg^{-1} daily. Recent work has shown that there is considerable interspecies variation in the dose rate required. Injectable preparations formulated for i.v. use are available in some countries and may be given intramuscularly. The dose for i.m. weekly administration is 75–100 mg kg^{-1}. Some formulations can cause severe muscle necrosis and should not be used for i.m. administration. An approved long-acting doxycycline injection is now available in the USA. Treatment should be continued for at least 45 days. Members of the tetracycline family of drugs tend to chelate with calcium thereby reducing the bioavailability of the doxycycline, hence dietary calcium levels should be limited and items such as cuttlefish and mineral blocks removed during therapy. Many birds treated in this way will require some antifungal therapy within the course of the treatment to avoid the consequence of enteric yeast infections.

Owners of confirmed chlamydial infection must be warned about the zoonotic potential of the infection and should be advised to consult their own physician. Owners should also be informed that there is no way of detecting whether their bird has been 'cured' of chlamydiosis by the end of the therapy. Follow up testing is recommended.

Many birds with chlamydiosis are immunosuppressed and should be evaluated for secondary bacterial and fungal infections which will require treatment. Care should include heat and fluid therapy, hepatoprotective therapy and paraimmunity inducers, as indicated.

221 i. As chicks age, their requirement for water in the diet decreases as does their tolerance of excessive water. Parents regulate water intake by feeding on food and water and allowing the mixture to settle in their crops. As the food settles, the food containing the most water is found in the top of the crop, more concentrated food at the bottom. Parents then feed chicks in order youngest to oldest. This allows younger chicks to receive more watery food then older ones.
ii. Excessive water intake in growing cockatiels has been found to result in over-hydration and emaciation. Chicks lack the capacity to excrete excess water and so are unable to ingest enough of the dilute diet to meet their requirements for total energy and for most essential nutrients. This condition usually results in crop stasis which is often confused with impaction. Frequently, breeders increase the amount of water in the diet to overcome suspected impactions rather than decreasing the dietary water content, which would allow the bird to meet its energy requirements.

222 A ten-year-old African grey parrot is presented to you with loss of voice, severe dyspnoea and a tracheal stridor. The diet of the bird consists of sunflower seeds and peanuts. The bird is not able to sit on its perch any more and the owner is afraid the bird will die from asphyxia. Which short-term and long-term treatment strategies are most likely to result in a successful outcome?

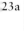

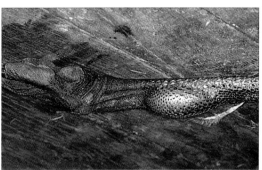

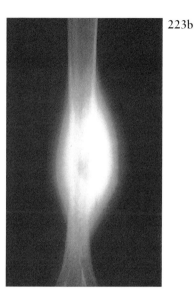

223 The photograph (**223a**) and radiograph (**223b**) are of an adult emu. Swelling of the tarso-metatarsal bone is evident, caused by periosteal proliferation as seen on the radiograph.
i. What is the cause?
ii. What is the treatment of choice and prognosis?

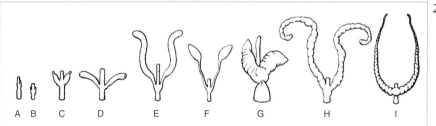

Intestinal caeca: (A) purple heron; (B) Eurasian sparrowhawk; (C) marabou stork; (D) rail; (E) helmeted guineafowl; (F) barn owl; (G) northern screamer; (H) great bustard; (I) ostrich

224 Caecae in birds (**224**) aid digestion of plant foods. They are most prominent in fowl and ostriches, in which they functionally resemble the caecum of horses.
i. What is the most important role of the caecae?
ii. Not all birds have functional caecae. Which group of birds lack a functional caecum?

161

222 The history and clinical signs are typical for an obstruction at the tracheal bifurcation. This can be metaplastic tissue caused by vitamin A deficiency or a fungal growth. Similar signs can be seen in smaller psittacines after inhalation of a foreign body, e.g. cockatiel with inhalation of millet seed. Immediate placement of the bird in an oxygen cage is indicated to stabilize the bird during the time that preparations are made for more definitive treatment.

When ready, the bird is masked down with isoflurane and an air sac tube is placed in a thoracic or the abdominal air sac to create an alternative, bypass, airway. After placing an air sac tube, a tracheoscopy is performed to visualize the obstruction. After the distance is established between the tracheal opening and the obstruction, attempts to remove it by suction can be made.

Postoperatively, intratracheal application of an aqueous antimycotic agent – e.g. miconazole or amphotericin B solution is started in conjunction with systemic antimycotic treatment. A multivitamin injection is given and the diet corrected. In the event that the obstruction cannot be removed by suction, the air sac tube can be left in place while a tracheotomy is performed at the level of, or as close as possible to, the tracheal lesion, and the foreign body removed via the incision.

Postoperatively, in-tracheal treatment with a soluble antimycotic should be given for five days after which repeat tracheoscopy should be performed to check for reformation. Local antimycotic treatment is given for at least five days or until the trachea is free of lesions. Systemic antimycotic treatment is continued for four weeks, or up to two months if aspergillosis is confirmed.

223 i. The cause of this presentation is trauma to the anterior aspect of the tarso-metatarsus causing a fracture and subsequent bone fragment sequestrum.
ii. The treatment of choice is surgery to remove the sequestered bone fragment. With proper postoperative care the affected area heals well with no long-term side effects.

224 i. The precise role of caecae in digestion remains unclear but it appears that bacteria in the caecae further digest and partially ferment digested foods into usable biochemical compounds that are absorbed through the caecal walls. Caecae may also function to separate the nutrient-rich fluid in partially digested food from the fibrous portion, which is eventually eliminated.
ii. Caecae are poorly developed or non-existent in most arboreal birds, e.g. psittacines and pigeons, perhaps because of the unacceptable weight of the watery, partially digested food in the intestine and the large structures required to handle it. Indeed, well-developed caecal fermentation is restricted to ground-dwelling as well as flightless birds, e.g. ratites, and is much more common in mammals than in birds.

225 An adult skua (*Cathar-acta skua*) was placed in an outdoor aviary after being housed in an indoor aviary for several years. The bird was presented with severe weakness and lethargy. The PCV was 18% (normal 35–55%).
i. Based upon the blood film (225), what is the most likely cause of the anaemia?
ii. How is this condition treated?

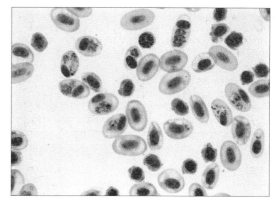
225

226 The carcass of a duck which has died acutely, with a haemorrhagic cloacal discharge is shown in 226. The breeder has had the same problem in three successive years, during April to June, with significant mortality in Muscovy ducks, Carolina (wood) ducks, blue-winged teal and mallard, but cranes and call ducks have not been affected.
i. What is the disease?
ii. What is the cause of the disease?

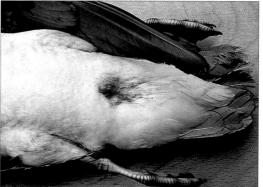
226

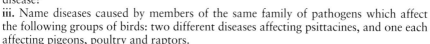

iii. Name diseases caused by members of the same family of pathogens which affect the following groups of birds: two different diseases affecting psittacines, and one each affecting pigeons, poultry and raptors.
iv. What are the biological properties of this family of pathogens and what effect do these properties have on the occurrence and control of the diseases?

225 i. The blood film demonstrates a marked number of immature erythrocytes suggestive of a marked regenerative response. Many of the erythrocytes contain intracytoplasmic inclusions that contain iron pigment and dramatically alter the position of the host cell nucleus. These inclusions are compatible with *Plasmodium* sp. gametocytes. Some strains of plasmodium are highly pathogenic resulting in a severe haemolytic anaemia (avian malaria).
ii. Chloroquine phosphate 10 mg kg^{-1} p.o. once then 5 mg kg^{-1} at 6, 18 and 24 hours – and primaquine phosphate 0.03 mg kg^{-1} p.o. daily for 3 days – are used in combination to treat avian malaria. Treatment with these and other anti-malarial drugs are often unrewarding and reinfections are common. Therefore, prevention by controlling the contact between birds and mosquito vectors is the best approach.

226 i. This is DVE ('duck plague').
ii. It is caused by a herpesvirus.
iii. Herpesviruses are responsible for:

- Pacheco's disease (caused by three separate serotypes of herpesvirus).
- Amazon tracheitis virus.
- Parakeet herpesvirus.
- Herpesvirus-associated, wart-like skin lesions (in cockatoos and macaws).
- Pigeon herpesvirus (causing IBH).
- Marek's disease (affecting poultry as well as other species).
- Falcon, eagle and owl herpesvirus.

iv. Herpesviruses are enveloped, tending to be well adapted to a particular species. The virus can survive for extended periods outside the body. In the case of DVE, the virus can survive in water for up to one month. Individual birds, which are not killed by the infections, tend to develop lifelong latent infections with periodic recrudescence. They replicate in and form intranuclear inclusion bodies. Spread may be vertical or horizontal. Infection can spread directly cell to cell within the body thereby avoiding circulating antibodies, leading to persistent infections. Herpesvirus vaccination will not currently prevent infection but will reduce the severity of infection. Vaccination will not prevent spread of virus. Acyclovir can be used successfully in infected birds – 10–40 mg kg^{-1} i.v. or s.c. t.i.d. – or as prophylaxis in the face of an outbreak at 80 mg kg^{-1} p.o. t.i.d. For the breeder who has recurrent outbreaks of infection, all surviving in-contact birds should be euthanased or isolated to prevent subsequent recontamination of the environment from time to time (especially at times of stress).

227 This is an ostrich faecal/urine sample (**227**).
i. What is the white substance within the urine portion of this sample?
ii. What is the presentation of ostrich faeces if the bird is suffering from a GI impaction?

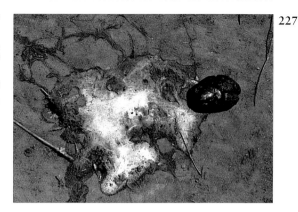

227

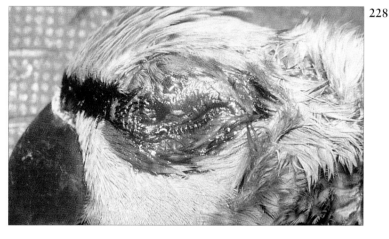

228

228 Shown in (**228**) is the presenting lesion in a bird from a group with several affected individuals.
i. What is your primary differential diagnosis?
ii. List several possible differential diagnoses.
iii. What is necessary to make a definitive diagnosis?
iv. How is the disease transmitted?

229 i. What are the sites for the placement of an intraosseous catheter?
ii. Describe the technique in each case.

227 i. These are uric acid crystals within the urine, a normal finding in most avian urine samples. Ostriches have a muscular sphincter between the urodeum and coprodeum, hence they are the only birds that can urinate independently of defecation.
ii. The presentation of ostrich faeces if impacted is scant, hard, dry pellets.

228 i. Poxvirus infection of the conjunctiva and periorbital skin.
ii. In psittacines, circovirus – PBFD – must also be considered as a similar lesion can be seen. In all birds, other infectious diseases, hypersensitivity, and trauma should be ruled out.
iii. A definitive diagnosis is made histologically by observing the characteristic intra-cytoplasmic – Bollinger – inclusion bodies in epithelial cells.
iv. The disease can spread by direct contact and by biting insects; control of the latter may be necessary to stop an outbreak.

229a

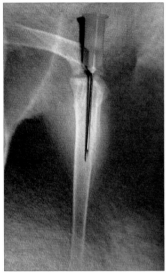

229

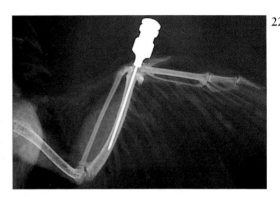

229 i. Cannulation of the distal ulna or proximal tibia, with a 20–25 gauge spinal needle, are the two most commonly recommended sites.
ii. Distal ulna – the carpal joint is flexed and after the feathers have been removed and the area aseptically prepared, the cannula is inserted into the distal end of the ulna, slightly ventral to the dorsal condyle, and the needle is rotated with gentle pressure until the cannula bores through the cortex into the marrow cavity (**229a**). By holding the ulna with one hand, the relationship and direction of the cannula to the bone can be established. Once the needle has been advanced into the medullary cavity, the stylet should be removed and a small amount of marrow aspirated to be sure the cannula is properly placed. The cannula should then be sutured in place.

Proximal tibia – after surgical preparation of the knee, the stifle is flexed and the cannula inserted into the tibial plateau of the tibial crest parallel to be tibia (**229b**). The catheter is inserted similarly to the ulna insertion and taped in position. It is essential to follow a strict aseptic technique.

230 A nine-year-old, yellow-naped Amazon was presented with lethargy and anorexia. On physical examination the clinician noted poor featheration and moderate pectoral muscle wasting. The droppings produced during the examination from the morning cage paper demonstrated polyuria. As part of an initial diagnostic and therapeutic plan, a blood panel was submitted.

AST: 230 IU l^{-1} (normal range 155–380 IU l^{-1})
LDH: 278 IU l^{-1} (normal range 160–360 IU l^{-1})
CK: 340 IU l^{-1} (normal range 120–410 IU l^{-1})
Bile acids: 560 µmol l^{-1} (normal range 35–144 µmol l^{-1})
Uric acid: 315 mmol l^{-1} (5.3 mg dl^{-1}) (normal range 137–583 mmol l^{-1} (2.3–9.8 mg dl^{-1}))

i. How would you interpret the results?
ii. What is the possible cause of the polyuria?

231 A pigeon loft owner reported multiple problems in his loft of racing pigeons, including birds with swollen hock or wing joints, increased numbers of dead-in-shells and clear eggs, mortality in young squabs and diarrhoea with marked weight loss. An occasional bird exhibited nervous signs such as twisting of the neck (**231**) and difficulty feeding.
i. What is the most likely diagnosis?
ii. How would you attempt to treat and control this disease?
iii. How would you differentiate this disease clinically from other causes of nervous disease in pigeons?

232 A client brought in some crusty material removed from the leg of his budgerigar. You examine this material under the microscope (**232**).
i. Identify the structures.
ii. Describe the treatment modalities.
iii. Describe prevention techniques.

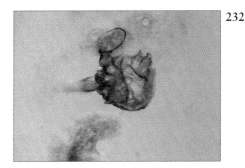

230 i. The enzymes are normal suggesting no current cellular damage and leakage from contributory sites including the liver, skeletal muscle, smooth muscle and cardiac muscle.

The bile acids are elevated, suggesting a reduced liver function associated with parenchymal changes. Previous liver damage has most likely occurred. The uric acid is normal, suggesting that the patient is not in terminal renal failure. However, uric acid is an insensitive indicator of avian renal function so kidney disease cannot be ruled out.
ii. In addition to renal disease, diabetes, mineral imbalances and polyuria are common presentations in birds with serious liver disease. The exact mechanism is not understood but is possibly related to the renal portal system which drains the liver and abdominal viscera.

231 i. The history and clinical signs are typical of salmonellosis, i.e. paratyphoid, usually involving *Salmonella typhimuritum* phage type 2 or 99.
ii. Treatment of all the birds in the loft with an antibacterial in the drinking water should be initiated. Suitable antibacterials include amoxycillin (1 g l⁻¹ of water for 7 days), combined trimethoprim and sulphamethoxazole (20 mg trimethoprim and 100 mg sulphamethoxazole per litre of water for 10 days) or enrofloxacin (200 mg l⁻¹ of water for 10 days).

The first course of antimicrobials may be unsuccessful in eliminating the organism from the flock and pooled faeces from the birds should be screened for *Salmonella* sp. following treatment, with the possibility of repeat medication. Medication should be combined with effective disinfection of the loft, feeders, drinkers, nest bowls, etc. Severely affected birds should be culled if no signs of improvement are seen. Control measures should aim to reduce the risks of *Salmonella* entering the loft, reduce the effects of the *Salmonella* should it gain entry to the loft, and should include loft monitoring for salmonellosis. The most likely source of *Salmonella* is another pigeon, so steps should be taken to prevent stray or feral pigeons entering. Good hygiene and avoiding overcrowding will reduce the subsequent spread of the organism. The use of an inactivated *Salmonella* vaccine has also been found to reduce spread in an infected loft. Strategic *Salmonella* monitoring of pooled loft faeces, prior to pairing up, should be part of the normal loft routine.
iii. Nervous signs may also be seen in pigeons that have been poisoned, for example by agricultural chemicals, α-chloralose or the therapeutic agent dimetridazole. The history of access to such poisons would help in such a diagnosis. However the most common condition to be considered in the differential diagnosis would be paramyxovirus 1 infection. In lofts with this infection there is usually a higher proportion of birds with diarrhoea and nervous signs than in lofts with salmonellosis and the diarrhoea with paramyxovirus is usually more watery. Loss of weight and appetite is more severe in cases of salmonellosis; swelling of the joints is a feature of salmonellosis, not paramyxovirus.

232 i. *Cnemidocoptes* sp. mite and egg.
ii. Ivermectin at 200 mg kg⁻¹ i.m.; repeat after 10 days if necessary.
iii. Treatment is usually curative. Identify, isolate and treat infected birds. It is often prudent to treat all in-contact birds as some infected birds may have very mild clinical signs.

233 At necropsy of a young amazon parrot the crop appeared as illustrated (233).
i. What is the most likely diagnosis and cause?
ii. What underlying factors should be considered in evaluating the lesion?

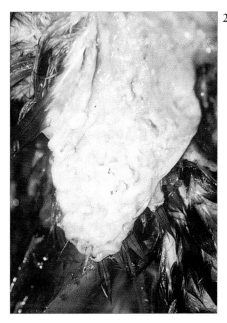

233

234 After plucking the contour feathers and down feathers from the ventral feather tract covering the pectoral region of a hawk (*Accipiter nisus*), small hair-like feathers have remained (234). What are they and what is their function?

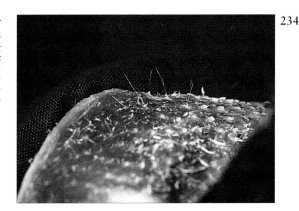

234

235 Haemochromatosis is a condition that affects a number of species of birds, including toucans; man may also be affected.
i. What effects may haemochromatosis have on man as compared to toucans?
ii. How does haemochromatosis differ in toucans and mynah birds?

233 i. Severe candidiasis – 'thrush' – due to *Candida albicans* or a similar species.
ii. This lesion is usually a secondary problem in a bird that is immunosuppressed. A complete necropsy and histological evaluation should be made with special attention to the bursa of Fabricius and other lymphoid organs.

234 These highly modified feathers – filoplumes – are not controlled by the muscle system that moves the position of all other feather types. The filoplume feather follicles are heavily endowed with nerve endings, suggesting that their function is sensory, ensuring that the bird is aware of the position of the rest of its feathers. Filoplumes are present in most species of bird.

235 i. In humans, there are two forms of haemochromatosis, primary and secondary. The primary, or idiopathic, form is a well-studied disease process. It is thought to be a recessively transmitted disorder, and is linked to the HLA region on the chromosome. It can be identified in affected individuals through a number of methods, including HLA genotyping. The genetic defect itself is thought to involve excessive absorption of iron by the mucosal cells of the intestinal tract although the exact nature of the defect is not known. It is not thought to be related to the amount of dietary iron as large amounts of available iron in the diet in non-affected individuals will not produce the disease. Iron may be abnormally deposited in a number of tissues including the liver, spleen, pancreas, thyroid gland, adrenal gland, the joints, the CNS and the heart. Disease processes directly related to this abnormal iron deposition include diabetes mellitus, altered liver function with a variety of hepatic dysfunction, and cardio-myopathy. The other form of haemochromatosis in humans is the secondary or acquired form. This is generally associated with chronic anaemia, a variety of haemo-lytic disorders and excessive iron absorption such as from exogenous iron adminis-tration. In comparison, in ramphastides, the vast majority of affected birds only have deposition of iron in the liver and clinically may demonstrate vague signs of disease or simply die.
ii. Haemochromatosis is clinically quite different in toucans and mynah birds. Indian Hill varieties (*Gracula religiosa*), Rothschild's mynah (otherwise known as Bali starling)(*Leucospar rothschildi*) have been affected to date. Clinical signs in these affected birds include a cachexic body condition, abdominal swelling due to ascites and/or hepatomegaly, and dyspnoea resulting from the ascites. Cardiomyopathy may also result from the disease process. Many affected mynahs have a history of chronic disease but some individuals have been observed to be acutely ill with death following shortly after observation of illness. It is not yet known whether the disease process of haemochromatosis in the affected mynahs is the same as in the toucans.

236 i. List the factors that cause death of eggs in each of the first, second and third trimesters.
ii. What levels of fertility and hatchability should be strived for?
iii. How often should eggs be turned during incubation?

237 A festiva Amazon (*Amazona a. festiva*) was presented with tail-bobbing and severe respiratory distress. Radiography and tracheoscopy give a considerable amount of additional clinical information and can be performed within seconds during recovery from anaesthesia. In this case, this structure (**237**) could be observed near the syrinx.
i. What is the diagnosis?
ii. How would you treat this bird?

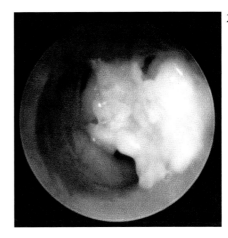

237

238 An adult, 279 g, yellow-naped Amazon parrot (*Amazona ochrocephala auropalliata*) was housed in a pet shop and developed a respiratory infection that was unsuccessfully treated for two weeks by the shop owner who used a variety of medications that were placed in the bird's drinking water. The bird was presented in a grave condition with a history of anorexia, weight loss, frequent regurgitation and loose droppings with green urates. Whole body radiographs revealed hepatomegaly and

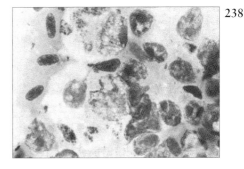

238

splenomegaly. The blood profile indicated a marked leucocytosis at 34.2×10^9 l^{-1} (N = 5–15×10^9 l^{-1}), heterophilia with toxic heterophils and a marked elevation in serum AST at 927 IU l^{-1} (N ≤ 175 IU l^{-1}) with a normal CK. The bird died within 2 hours of presentation. A gross necropsy revealed a marked reduction of the pectoral muscle mass, a sinusitis, cloudy air sacs, hepatomegaly and splenomegaly.
i. Based upon the cytological findings from the Wright's-stained liver imprint (**238**), what is the most likely cause of illness and death?
ii. What special stains could be used to confirm the diagnosis?

236 i. First trimester:

- Contaminated eggs.
- Poor egg handling or storage.
- Poor incubation (temperature; humidity; lack of turning).
- Genetic abnormalities (inbreeding).
- Breached integrity of the eggshell.
- Transovarian or postlaying infection of the egg.
- Drug or pesticide effects on the egg.

Second trimester:

- Genetic abnormalities (inbreeding).
- Parental nutritional deficiencies or imbalances.
- Infections (bacterial, viral or fungal).
- Poor incubation (temperature; humidity; lack of turning).
- Poor egg handling in the first trimester.

Third trimester:

- Incubation faults (temperature; humidity; lack of turning).
- Brooder faults (temperature; humidity; lack of turning).
- Infections.
- Malpositioning prior to hatching.
- Parental nutritional deficiencies.
- Genetic abnormalities.
- Poor hatchery hygiene.

ii. Fertility and hatchability levels vary greatly between species and individuals. Fertility tends to be lower in inbred, older or younger birds, and at the beginning and end of each breeding season. The breeder should try to achieve 85–95% fertility. Hatchability is also variable with respect to the species and the above factors; the breeder should aim for 80–85%.

iii. Most eggs are positioned on their side with the round (air sac) end slightly elevated. Eggs should be turned 6 to 12 times daily – each turn being between 30–45° or the eggs may be turned along the longitudinal axis. The first trimester is the most crucial period for egg turning; failure to turn in this period will usually lead to disaster. If a chick appears to be developing slowly, increasing the turns is thought to be of assistance in some cases.

237 i. This mycotic granuloma within the trachea is most often caused by *Aspergillus* sp.

ii. Specific antimycotic treatment – amphotericin; itraconazole; ketoconazole – as well as symptomatic treatment – fluids; vitamin A; tube feeding – has to be performed. Because of severe respiratory distress, in many cases an abdominal air sac tube should be used; surgical removal of the granuloma can also be performed. This is often the only sign of systemic fungal infection.

238 i. The liver imprint reveals macrophages with small, round, basophilic, intracytoplasmic inclusions that are compatible with those of *Chlamydia psittaci*.

ii. Gimenez and Macchiavello's stains can be used to confirm the presence of chlamydial inclusions in cytological specimens.

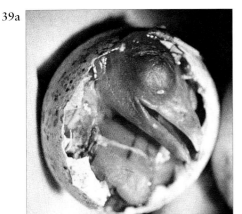
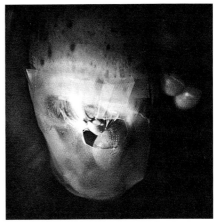

239 Malpositioned embryos are shown in **239a, b**.
i. Using the traditional system, classify the malposition and give a short description.
ii. Describe the effect each of the seven types of malpositioning can have on hatching death.

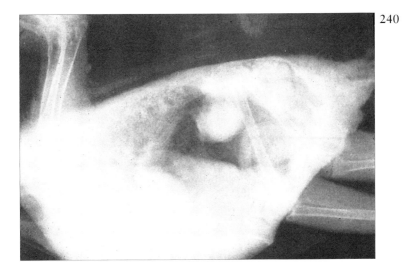

240 i. What is remarkable in this radiograph (**240**)? Describe what you see.
ii. What clinical signs are to be expected with each of the differential diagnosis?
iii. How would you confirm your diagnosis?

239 i. 239a represents malposition 6 (the head over the right wing); **239b** shows malposition 2 (the head is in the small end of the egg at hatch).
ii. The seven types of malposition are as follows:

- Malposition 1 – the embryo's head is found between the thighs; this is a normal position early in incubation. However, during the last third of incubation, the embryo should move its head up and under the right wing. Malposition 1 is always fatal; it can be associated with above normal incubation temperatures.
- Malposition 2 – the embryo's head is located in the small end of the egg, as in **239b**. The position is lethal in 50% of cases. Assistance in hatching improves the hatching success rate.
- Malposition 3 – this occurs when the chick rotates its head under the left wing instead of the right. This malposition is nearly always lethal and is associated with malnutrition in laying females, high incubation temperatures or improper positioning of the egg during incubation.
- Malposition 4 – the body is rotated in the long axis of the egg. The head is, therefore, away from the air cell and along the side of the egg. Without assistance, this malposition is often fatal as the embryo never breaks through to breathe.
- Malposition 5 – this occurs when the feet are located over the head. Because of this malposition, the legs are not located properly to kick and cause the body to rotate as the chick is cutting out. Unless hatching is assisted, the results will often prove fatal.
- Malposition 6 – the head is over rather than under the right wing, as in **239a**. This can still result in a live hatch with few complications.
- Malposition 7 – this occurs when the embryo is small or the egg is spherical. The embryo is found lying crosswise in the egg instead of in the normal orientation with the head up near the air cell. This malposition is often fatal.

240 i. The radiograph shows a focal density of soft tissue in the cranial kidney area. The most likely differentials are an active testis, an aspergilloma, a neoplastic mass or a mycobacterial granuloma.
ii. A bird with an active testicle would be expected to be in good body condition. It has been reported by owners that occasionally birds with physiological testicular hypertrophy may show lameness or slight respiratory distress. Space-occupying hypertrophy can compromise the respiratory system. An enlarged testicle may cause lameness by exertion of pressure on the pelvic nerves.

A patient with an aspergillomata of this size will often present with respiratory distress, anorexia, regurgitation, weight loss and lethargy.

A bird with mycobacteriosis or a neoplastic mass in this site would be expected to show dyspnoea and weight loss, often in the absence of anorexia.
iii. A CBC can be used; abnormalities would exclude a physiological testicular hypertrophy.

Exploratory endoscopy with biopsy should be considered to be the most useful diagnostic method. A fungal culture can be attempted but is not always successful as aspergillotic infections can be localized and encapsulated and hence difficult to access. ELISA tests, as an accurate diagnostic tool for aspergillosis, are not available in many countries. Demonstrating acid-fast rods in tissue sections is currently the preferred method for mycobacterial diagnosis. Biopsy can differentiate between neoplasia and mycobacteriosis.

241 What are possible causes of iron storage disease in toucans?

242 A fledgeling black-throated laughing thrush was found dead on the cage floor. This bird had fledged several weeks earlier and was recently moved, along with a sibling, to a separate cage from the parent birds because the parents were starting a second clutch. The bird exhibited no clinical signs of illness prior to its death. The cage mate, a sibling, was showing no clinical signs of illness. A gross necropsy was performed and revealed hepato-

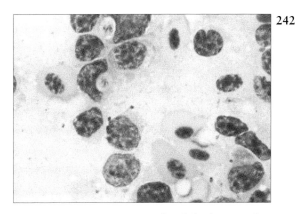

megaly and splenomegaly. Contact smears (imprints) were made of the lungs, spleen and liver. The cytologic finding in a splenic imprint is shown (**242**).
i. What is the cytodiagnosis?
ii. How is this disease treated in birds?

243 Illustrated in **243** is a rarely seen form of which disorder commonly seen in macaws and Amazon parrots?

- *Cnemidocoptes* mite infestation.
- Papillomatosis.
- Squamous cell carcinoma.
- Hyperkeratosis of the skin associated with ageing and vitamin A deficiency.

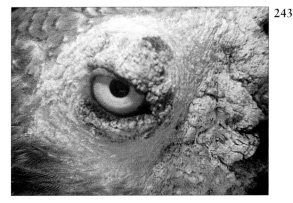

241 Possible causes for iron storage disease in affected avian species can only be speculated at present. The manifestation of disease and the aetiology in the variety of avian species may be similar but probably varies, as do the clinical signs and the disease itself in these birds. A list of possible causes for iron storage disease in toucans includes:

- An inherited metabolic defect in the mucosal lining of the small intestine, thus allowing for the abnormal absorption and processing of dietary iron.
- Presence or past presence of an infectious agent that enables the intestinal lining to absorb more dietary iron with subsequent deposition in the liver. This might include viral or parasitic agents.
- Unknown metabolic factors that may allow the excessive absorption of dietary iron.
- Excessive dietary iron – though not the primary cause – may be significant in the development and manifestation of iron storage disease. There may be complex interactions involving dietary components such as deficiencies of certain essential amino acids, vitamins and imbalances in dietary mineral composition. There is also some concern that ascorbic acid in the diet of susceptible species may potentially enhance the bioavailability and thus the absorption of dietary iron.
- Some theories revolve around the concept that tannins or tannic acid (naturally occurring compounds in certain trees) may somehow allow for a protective relationship involving the natural chelation of iron, and thus reduce its absorption. Tannins are thought to be naturally deposited in tropical river waters where free-living ramphastides drink. This theory assumes that these tannins act as a natural counter to iron overload in susceptible species.
- One assumption presumes that there is a relationship between the development of haemochromatosis and stress. This theory suggests that stresses such as breeding, captivity and environmental influences lead to the increased and abnormal storage of iron in those susceptible species.
- Lastly, a completely idiopathic cause is plausible.

242 i. Numerous lymphocytes, and two lymphocytes with intracytoplasmic inclusions, are visible in **242**. The oval inclusions stain poorly, have pink-staining chromatin and indent the lymphocyte nucleus creating a crescent shape to the nucleus. The inclusions are compatible with sporozoites of *Atoxoplasma* sp., such as *A. serini*.
ii. There is no effective treatment for atoxoplasmosis described for birds. Sulpha drugs have been suggested as a treatment. Sulphachloro-pyrazine may decrease the shedding of oocysts. Primaquine has been suggested to suppress the tissue form of the parasite.

243 This parrot was found to have these skin lesions shortly after importation. Histopathology revealed lesions of cutaneous papillomatosis, and virus particles consistent with *Papillomavirus* were found on electron microscopy. This bird did not have oral or cloacal lesions. These lesions continued for years despite numerous attempts at therapy and the bird was ultimately euthanased due to the severity of the lesions.

244 The photomicrograph (**244**) shows a tuberculous granuloma in a section of the liver of a duck. In waterfowl infected with avian tuberculosis:

i. Is there any intersex differential rate of incidence?

ii. Does the disease have implications for staff or visitors to the collection?

iii. List at least three methods of making ante-mortem diagnosis.

iv. What measures can be taken to reduce or prevent the incidence within a collection?

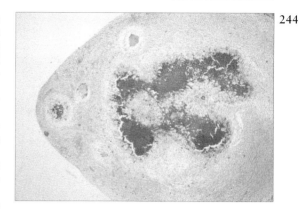

244

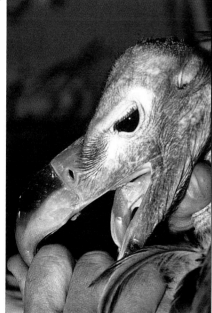

45a

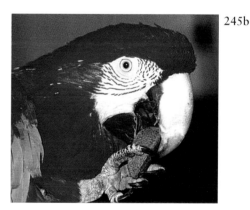

245b

245 Head of a falconiform compared with psittaciform craniofacial hinge. What is the anatomical difference between birds, exemplified by this vulture (*Aegypius tracheliotus*) (**245a**) and the Psittaciforme family (**245b**) when it comes to increasing the size of their gape – prokinesis – and using their beak to prehend their food?

244 i. Both sexes show a similar incidence rate although there is a variable seasonality in clinical disease. Both sexes show considerable disease following the rigours of the winter, although female birds also demonstrate a considerable increase in incidence following the stress of the breeding season.

ii. *Mycobacterium avium* is a human pathogen, hence the handling and treatment of affected cases carries a zoonotic risk, as does heavy environmental contamination. The disease now shows a greatly increased zoonotic prevalence, particularly in humans infected with HIV or suffering other immune suppressive diseases. However, current research indicates that the serotype affecting humans may be different from that affecting birds. This field requires considerable research input as different species of bird tend to be affected by different serotypes, hence there may yet be a connection.

iii. WBC counts are generally in excess of 8×10^9 l^{-1}; heterophilia, monocytosis and fibrinogen levels will be raised typically above 6 (N = 4 g l^{-1}), frequently with a hypochromic, microcytic anaemia. It has been shown that these changes do not occur until the disease has progressed considerably. Intradermal skin testing is not reliable.

Whole blood agglutination testing has been used, although results are not consistent. Faecal culture is unreliable due to the length of time required and false positive results; faecal examination for acid-fast organisms also gives rise to many false positives. An ELISA test for waterfowl has been developed at the Wildfowl and Wetlands Trust, Slimbridge, UK, although it is still not reliable for some stiff-tail ducks, geese and swans. However, this test has a great future potential. If disease is suspected on clinical signs, chronic weight loss, green droppings, lethargy, lameness, etc., disease can often be confirmed by endoscopic examination of the liver. Tubercles can be found at any site in the body, though most cases will demonstrate small white foci in the liver.

iv. The measures are: (1) screening of birds prior to joining the collection; (2) new introductions should be young birds, reared on clean ground; (3) control of feral birds who might contaminate the environment; (4) post-mortems of all deaths; (5) minimizing wet areas around the water's edge (by concreting); (6) if a number of ponds exist, each should have a clean water supply; contaminated water from one pond should not feed another; (7) vaccination of young birds with *M. vacci*, if available; (8) screening of collection and elimination of positive birds to reduce environmental contamination; (9) removal of excessive vegetation from around ponds will reduce tubercle survival time in the environment.

245c

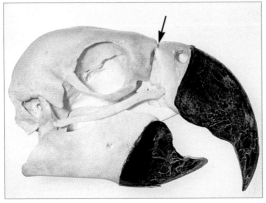

245 The majority of birds have elastic zones at the junction of the maxilla and the frontal bone or within the upper jaw itself. Only psittacine birds, e.g. *Ara* sp., have a synovial joint – the craniofacial hinge (arrowed) – that allows greater and stronger movements of the upper jaw relative to the lower jaw (**245c**).

246 Iron storage disease is the result of the storage of excess iron in soft tissues, particularly the spleen and liver. At high levels this results in damage to either the morphology or function of the tissue.
i. Is diet a significant cause of iron storage disease?
ii. What part does physiological stress play in iron storage disease?

247 Post-mortem examination of a four-month-old pigeon revealed a greatly enlarged liver with some perihepatitis (**247**). *E.coli* was isolated from the viscera. Prior to death the bird appeared hunched up, had diarrhoea, and died after 48 hours. Other lesions observed in the live bird were yellowish plaques adherent to the mucosa of the tongue and pharynx.
i. What is your diagnosis and how would you confirm it?
ii. Other than salmonellosis, what other condition may commonly result in a swollen liver, often with a swollen spleen, in young birds with diarrhoea?
iii. How would you treat and control these two conditions?

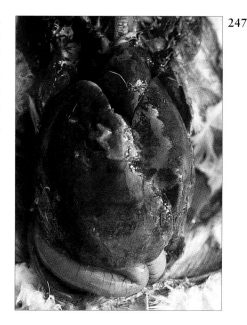

247

248 After induction of anaesthesia in a hornbill (*Anthracoceros malayanus*), the anaesthetist had difficulty inserting an endotracheal tube into the larynx because of the structure illustrated (**248**). Is this a normal anatomical structure and, if so, what is it? Is a similar structure seen in any other species or family?

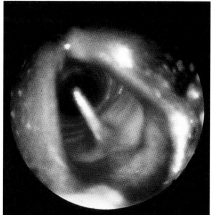

248

246 i. The typical pet bird diet is unlikely to be the cause of iron storage disease. Most birds are exposed to levels of iron in the diet that are far in excess of the levels required to maintain iron stores. To get to lower levels requires chemical treatment of food to remove the iron, yet most birds live many years without succumbing to iron storage disease.

ii. Recent evidence indicates that iron storage disease is a result, in part, of stress. Stress hormones increase the levels of some proteins important in the transport of iron. When these proteins are increased by stress, iron stores are also increased. One important factor in iron storage disease is stress reduction in the affected, or potentially affected, bird. Some stresses that have been shown to increase the storage of iron or other minerals in soft tissues include toxic stress, immunological stress and starvation followed by refeeding.

247 i. The combination of yellow plaques in the mouth, diarrhoea, death and hepatomegaly at post-mortem examination is strongly suggestive of an IBH caused by a herpes- or adenovirus. Frequently there are concurrent infections such as with *E. coli*, *Candida albicans*, *Trichomonas*, *Hexamita*, *Chlamydia*, *Coccidia* and pigeon pox. Diagnosis is confirmed by histopathological examination of the liver in which will be found liver cell necrosis and the presence of intranuclear inclusion bodies. In cases of IBH caused by a herpesvirus, eosinophilic intranuclear inclusion bodies predominate while basophilic inclusions are commoner if the IBH results from an adenovirus infection. Virus isolation or demonstration may be attempted to determine the exact nature of the virus.

ii. Other than salmonellosis, chlamydiosis should be considered as a possible cause of hepatomegaly and splenomegaly in young pigeons with diarrhoea. Although usually thought of as a cause of respiratory disease in conjunction with other organisms, *Chlamydia psittaci* is also a relatively common cause of watery diarrhoea in young pigeons. Chlamydia antigen may be detected by PCR or ELISA, although false positives may occur using the latter test, especially if faeces are tested; alternatively, paired serological samples may be examined.

iii. There is no specific treatment for IBH but any concurrent loft problems should be identified and treated. If chlamydiosis is diagnosed, treatment of all birds in the loft with tetracyclines in the drinking water is recommended; also, the fancier should be made aware of the possible zoonotic nature of this disease. Supportive treatment in the form of electrolytes may be beneficial in both conditions. Adult birds may become symptomless carriers of *Chlamydia psittaci*, herpesvirus IBH, and possibly adenovirus IBH, passing on the infection to the young birds in the loft, which may then develop clinical disease. Alternatively, the young birds may pick up the organism from young birds from other lofts during transportation, etc. Control measures should therefore be aimed at limiting the effects of these organisms in the young birds by the control of concurrent pathogens, good hygiene and by reducing stress in the young birds to a minimum.

248 This is the ventral crest – *crista ventralis* – of the larynx. It has been described in penguins (Spheniscidae), *Anas* and *Apteryx*. It may also be seen in other species such as certain hornbills, toucans and gulls.

249 i. What are the two most likely causes of bacterial arthritis in racing pigeons?
ii. What is the differential diagnosis for a swelling in the region of the elbow joint in this species (**249**)?
iii. How would you confirm your tentative diagnosis?
iv. What would be the treatment of choice for the two diseases indicated?

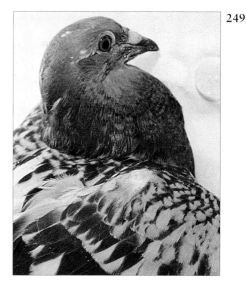

249

250 This Amazon parrot presented with acute diarrhoea and disturbance of balance (**250**).
i. What is your diagnosis from this radiograph?
ii. What clinical signs would be expected?
iii. What are the commonest errors that may result in a clinician failing to make the correct diagnosis?

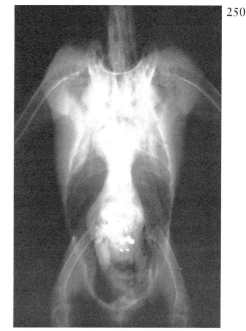

250

249 i. *Salmonella typhimurium* var. *kopenhagen* and *Streptococcus bovis*. Arthritis of the elbow joint is pathognomonic for salmonellosis in racing pigeons.
ii. Fracture, luxation, haematoma, tumour and feather cyst. Other clinical signs seen in other birds in the loft may include torticollis, diarrhoea, skin abscesses, infertile eggs and mortality.
iii. Diagnosis can be made by culture of a pooled faecal sample from the loft or by serological examination when pigeons are not vaccinated. Synovial culture of the elbow joint is often disappointing.
iv. Treat the whole flock with trimethoprim and sulphamethoxazole at 50 and 10 mg kg^{-1} per day respectively. Consider the use of an inactivated vaccine for future prevention. *Streptococcus bovis* is widespread in asymptomatic pigeons – facultative pathogen – but may cause lameness of the wings – tenosynovitis of *M. supracoracoideus* – or legs, emaciation, green slimy excreta, palpable areas of necrosis in the pectoral muscle, meningitis and septicaemia. Isolation needs special conditions: enrichment medium and Slanetz and Bartley agar. The recommended treatment in cases with both clinical signs and isolation of *S. bovis* is ampicillin at 175 mg kg^{-1} per day (2 g l^{-1} drinking water) for 5 days.

250 i. There are metal particles detectable in the digestive tract. In the majority of cases these are lead, which causes typical signs of heavy metal toxicity. Zinc particles are also common, especially when birds are housed in new galvanized cages or old ones that have been soldered.
ii. In companion birds, one most often sees an acute course in lead intoxication. In free-ranging birds, chronically diseased individuals are most frequently seen by the veterinarian. In an acute case, the clinical signs classically occur within 48 hours of ingestion – these may include depression, lethargy, weakness, anorexia, regurgitation (which develops into severe vomiting), polyuria and diarrhoea. The faeces may be extremely green or contain large amounts of blood. In addition, any disorders of the CNS – tremors; ataxia; even blindness – may be seen.
iii. Failure to radiograph such a case is a common error. A bird presenting with any of these signs should always be radiographed even if the owner insists that the bird could not have ingested lead. Another error would be the misinterpretation of poor quality radiographs. Ventricular heavy metal fragments must not be mistaken for grit.

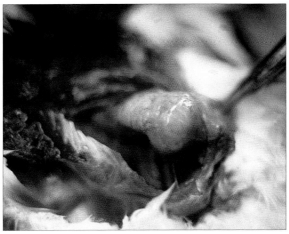

251a

251 A budgerigar fancier has had a small proportion of his birds losing weight and dying over the last two months. A few of the diseased birds vomit and some have diarrhoea. Post-mortem examination of one bird shows enlargement and pallor of the proventriculus (251a, b). What is the condition likely to be? How may the disease be diagnosed, in life and after death? What treatment, if any, can be given?

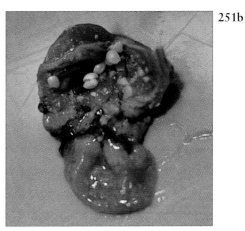

251b

252 List eleven factors which are likely to affect the fertility of a pair of birds.

251, 252: Answers

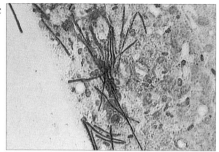

251c

251 As a number of birds are affected, the condition is likely to be megabacteriosis (**251c**). Other causes of proventricular dilation are likely to affect only individual birds at any one time. Care must be taken in diagnosing flock problems from a single post-mortem examination as the bird examined may not be typical of the problem. Diagnosis in life depends on the demonstration of the organism in crop washes or faeces but the number of organisms in these sites may be small. There is no way of distinguishing the carrier state from the clinical disease except on the basis of the symptoms, but the bird could be ill due to another disease. After death, a post-mortem examination will reveal proventricular dilatation, a degree of thickening at the proventriculus–ventriculus junction, often with ulceration. There is an excess of mucus in the otherwise usually empty proventriculus and Gram-stained films of this mucus will reveal the organisms in large numbers. The contents of the proventriculus will be about pH neutral instead of the normal pH of 0.7–2 since affected birds do not produce hydrochloric acid. A 10 day course of a high dose – 0.5 mg per budgerigar – of amphotericin B given orally at least twice a day will eliminate the organism, but about half the birds will not recover clinically due to residual proventricular damage. Acidification of the drinking water with hydrochloric, citric or acetic acid is said to work but often the birds will not drink sufficiently acidified water to be effective. Megabacteriosis is extremely common in exhibition budgerigars in the UK.

252 Factors likely to affect the fertility of a pair of birds are:

1 First, that the pair are of the opposite sex, same species and are sexually mature.
2 Environment – day length, climate, season. Some birds of the same species but which originate from geographically different areas will continue to come into breeding condition at different times, thereby preventing successful breeding.
3 Pair bonding – many breeders believe that certain pairs are unsuited and will not bond, while if separated, they will each breed quite happily with alternative mates. Other breeders believe that this situation only arises if the breeding conditions were unsuitable in some respect. Hand-reared birds of certain species do not mate readily with those of their own kind. Psittacines are generally not affected in this way.
4 Human interference may prevent successful breeding.
5 Nest materials, boxes and nest box holes may act as an essential stimulus for breeding.
6 Previous reproductive experience tends to reduce the requirement for environmental stimulation and hence helps in future breeding success.
7 Nutrition Ca, Na, energy, and vitamins A, D and E are all particularly important.
8 Physical (in)ability to copulate.
9 Physiologically normal reproductive organs in both birds.
10 Concurrent disease.
11 Antibiotic usage.

253 Pneumatized medullary cavity of the femur (253). The femur of a Eurasian buzzard (*Buteo buteo*) has been opened to show the medullary cavity. Why and how is this bone modified in comparison with the same bone in mammals?

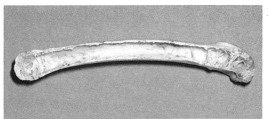

253

254 Burns are not uncommon in avian medicine. Most common burns result from contact with hot liquids, water (scalds) or cooking oil, electrical burns from chewing on electrical wires and from being fed hot formula in preweaning birds. Burns resulting from entrapment in burning buildings or inside containers (chick incubators with burning bedding) are not as common but are much more difficult to treat with the complication of smoke inhalation. How are burns classified in the avian patient and why is this classification important in therapy?

• Burns are best classified as sterile or infected to determine the need for anti-infective therapy.
• Burns are best classified as sub-acute, acute, and chronic to determine the need for bandaging.
• Burns are best classified as thermal or chemical to determine the need for topical therapy of chemical substances.
• Burns are best classified by their severity as superficial, partial thickness or full thickness to determine the degree of tissue involvement.

255 A pair of rose-breasted cockatoos are presented (255) with a history of infertility during the last breeding season. The breeder reports that the birds do not seem as active lately and today noticed some digested blood in one of the bird's droppings.
i. What additional history would be useful?
ii. What diagnostic tests would be useful?
iii. What would be the best treatment or prevention for the current problem?

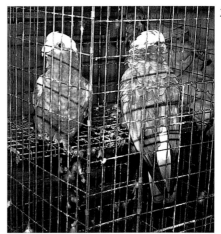

255

253 The cortex is thinner and more brittle than in a mammal. The avian cortex is supported by a network of fine bony trabeculae which give added strength to the cortex. The medullary cavity is pneumatized via the trochanteric fossa in the cranial diaphysis which connects with the abdominal air sac. All these modifications allow the femur to remain strong but with a decreased weight when compared with the femur of a mammal, in order to reduce the energy required for flight.

254 The burns of avian patients are best classified by their severity (as in the last choice). Superficial burns – where only the epidermis is affected – result in transient erythema and desquamation of the epidermis; the site is hyperaesthetic. Clinical signs include hyperaemia, desquamation and pain. Partial thickness burns are those where the burn depth extends to the mid-dermis. Loss of epidermis is complete, capillaries and venules in the dermis are dilated and congested and they exude plasma. The site may be painful – especially feet, legs and facial skin – but sensitivity is decreased. Clinical signs include exudation, pain and decreased sensitivity. Change in ease of feather pulling – as noted with hair in mammals – may not be affected due to the depth of the feather follicle. Full thickness burns result in coagulation of the epidermis and dermis so that they are no longer vital. Severe oedema of the subcutis develops from the increased permeability of deep vessels, and necrosis of the damaged tissues occurs resulting in dry, leathery eschar. Feathers may be easily pulled if the burn is deep and scaled skin may peel easily. Clinical signs include necrotic tissue without sensation, subcutaneous oedema, little or no pain and feathers that are easily pulled.

255 i. Additional history should include:

- Have the birds been reproductively successful in the past?
- Are there any other birds in the same aviary with the same signs?
- Have there been any changes in the birds' environment or diet in the last year?

The owner reports that the birds have been moved into a new breeding cage that the owner had made out of galvanized wire.

ii. Based on clinical signs and the potential exposure to galvanized wire, the following tests should be run:

- CBC/chemistry profile.
- Faecal examination and culture.
- Blood lead and zinc analysis (blood must not be collected in rubber-topped containers).
- Radiographs.
- Chlamydia titres.

iii. The diagnostics revealed abnormally high blood zinc levels in both birds (greater than 800 mg dl^{-1} or 8 ppm). The melena reported in the history was most likely due to necrotizing ventriculitis which is a common sequel to zinc toxicity. Treatment involves removal of the birds from their accommodation as well as the administration of Ca-EDTA at 35 mg kg^{-1} i.m. b.i.d. for 7 days). DMSA is now preferred for the treatment of lead and zinc poisoning as it is safer than CaEDTA. Dose DMSA at 30 mg kg^{-1} for 10 days or for 5 days per week for 3–5 weeks. No metallic particles were seen on the radiographs.

Index

eyes (*continued*)
  lens 158, 217
  lens subluxation 176
  retrobulbar mass 169
  ulcerative keratitis 95

faecal flotation 80
Falco cherrug 2
fat, dietary 60
fatty liver 204
feather cysts 124
feather discoloration 97, 101
'feather duster' 41
feather dystrophy 89
feather pulp haemorrhage 10
feathers 10
  achromatosis 101
  budgerigar fledgeling disease 84
  burns and 254
  exudative folliculitis 89
  filoplumes 234
  functions of 1
  and malnutrition 97
  and oil toxicosis 122
  parasitic loss of 205
  plucking of, causes 198
  polyfollicular lesions 35
  preening 71
  and sexual frustration 11
  and stress bars 210
  and surgery 46
  traumatic loss of 205
  types of 1
  see also psittacine beak and feather
    disease (PBFD)
femoral nerve 138
femur, pneumatized medullary cavity 252
fenbendazole 80
fertility 252
fibrogranulomatous lesions 177
filarial worms 2
filoplumes 1, 234
fires 254
  and intoxication 79
fistula, crop 128
fledgeling disease 84
flight 113, 180
  energy for 116
flock density 110
fluconazole 22
fluid therapy 28
forceps, for microsurgery 98
foreign bodies 173, 177, 222
  in the crop 75

foreign bodies (*continued*)
  proventricular 100
fractures 106, 164
  multiple 211
  wild birds 202
free fatty acids 157
'fret marks' 210
frostbite 206

gangrene, dry 206
gapeworm 32
gaseous anaesthesia 43, 99
  reflexes and 144
gastrointestinal candidiasis 22
Giardia sp. 143
Gimenez–Macchiavello stains 238
glucocorticoids 64
glue, for maxillary fractures 106
gout 139, 155, 167
granular conjunctivitis 181
grass, proventricular impaction with 50
gut bleeding 201

haemochromatosis 9, 30, 63, 145, 160,
    171, 213, 235, 241, 246
haematozoal infections 166
haemolytic anaemia 225
Haemoproteus spp. 67
haemorrhages 10, 23
haemorrhagic enteritis 91, 201
haloperidol 11
halothane 46, 99
head loupes 217
head louse, human 56
head trauma 64
heart rate, in anaesthesia 114
heavy metal poisoning 5, 8, 208
hepatic encephalopathy 8
hepatitis 74, 112
hernia, abdominal wall 47
herpesvirus 112, 142, 225
hetastarch 14
heterophils, toxic 203
Histomonas meleagrides 18, 174
hobby loupes 217
hormones, sex 11
human-to-avian infections 56, 57
  head louse 56
  psittacosis 57
human chorionic gonadotrophin 11
human head louse 56
'humpback' 120
'hunger traces' 210
hydrocortisone 64

ostrich pox 81
oviduct 132
   prolapse 59
oxygen absorption 103, 163
   air sacs 96

Pacheco's disease 112, 225
pain control 136
papillomas 191
papillomavirus 118, 243
paramyxovirus 1 infections 55, 200
parathyroid gland hyperplasia 126
pecten 37, 95
Pediculus humanus var. *capitus* 56
D-penicillamine 5
peritonitis, egg-related 76
pesticides 8, 31
phallus
   ostrich 20
   prolapse 59
pheasant coronavirus nephritis 36
pigeons
   carcasses of 183
   feeding 183
   housing 72
   poisoning of 231
   quality of 40
   as raptor feed 183
   segregation of 147
   selection, by fanciers 212
   squabs 80
   stocking density 110
piperacillin 119, 218
pituitary gland adenoma 44
plantar granulomas 177
plant chewing 54
Plasmodium sp. 159, 225
pneumatized medullary cavity, femur 253
pneumonia 192
polyfollicular lesions 35
polyomavirus infection 10, 84
polyuria 73
post-traumatic epistaxis 23
poxvirus infection 19, 81, 228
praziquantel 91
prednisolone 64
preen gland 199
preening 71
primaquine 225
probenecid 139
professional opinions 122
progesterone 11
prolapses 59, 68
propatagium 113

prostaglandin E_2 24
protein, dietary 51, 97, 204
proventricular dilation syndrome 66, 184, 188
proventricular foreign bodies 100
proventricular grass impaction 50
proventriculotomy 38, 100
proventriculus, surgery 219
Prozac 11
Pseudomonas aeruginosa 119
Pseudomonas sp. 145
pseudo-tuberculosis 187, 194
psittacine beak and feather disease (PBFD) 12, 84, 228
psittacine proventricular dilation syndrome (PPDS) 184
psittacosis 52, 154
   from humans 57
   see also chlamydiosis
pyrantel pamoate 140
pyrethrin 93, 97
pyrimethamine 215

raccoons 207
radiosurgical incision 141
red blood cells 67, 225
   and lead poisoning 208
'renal gout' 201
respiration 96, 163, 172, 173
   in anaesthesia 114, 144
respiratory disease, progressive 111
respiratory rate, in anaesthesia 114, 144
respiratory system 108
retina 37
retrobulbar masses 169
riboflavin deficiency 101
rickets, rib 190
Ringer's solution 14
rodenticides 82
Romonowsky stains 39
ronidazole 15, 80, 143
rotaviruses 87
roundworm 140

salmonellosis 18, 178, 194, 200, 231, 249
salt secreting gland 209
Sarcocystis falcatula 134
sarcocystosis 134
scaly leg 64
scissor beak deformity 161
second opinion 122
'segmental feather dystrophy' 210
semen sampling 78
semiplumes 1

For Reference

Not to be taken from this room

WITHDRAWN